# HEARING-HANDICAPPED ADULTS

REMEDIATION OF COMMUNICATION DISORDERS
SERIES
Frederick N. Martin, Series Editor

STUTTERING

———————————————————— Edward G. Conture

HEARING IMPAIRMENTS IN YOUNG CHILDREN

———————————————————— Arthur Boothroyd

HARD OF HEARING CHILDREN IN REGULAR SCHOOLS

Mark Ross with Diane Brackett
———————————————— and Antonia Maxon

HEARING-HANDICAPPED ADULTS

———————————————————— Thomas G. Giolas

ACQUIRED NEUROGENIC DISORDERS

———————————————————— Thomas P. Marquardt

LANGUAGE DISORDERS IN PRESCHOOL CHILDREN

———————————————————— Patricia R. Cole

LANGUAGE DISORDERS IN SCHOOL AGE CHILDREN

———————————————————— Mary Lovey Wood

Forthcoming

ARTICULATION DISORDERS

———————————————————— Ronald K. Sommers

CEREBRAL PALSY

———————————————————— James C. Hardy

Thomas G. Giolas

*University of Connecticut*

# HEARING-HANDICAPPED ADULTS

Prentice-Hall, Inc., Englewood Cliffs, New Jersey 07632

*Library of Congress Cataloging in Publication Data*

GIOLAS, THOMAS G.
   Hearing-handicapped adults.
   (Remediation of communication disorders)
   Bibliography: p.
   Includes index.
   1. Hearing impaired.   2. Hearing impaired—
Rehabilitation.   I. Title.   II. Series.
HV2380.G56        362.4'2        81-13897
ISBN 0-13-384693-8        AACR2

Printed in the United States of America

10  9  8  7  6  5  4  3  2  1

Editorial/production supervision by Virginia Cavanagh Neri
Interior design by Maureen Olsen
Cover design by Maureen Olsen
Manufacturing buyer: Edmund W. Leone

ISBN 0-13-384693-8

Prentice-Hall International, Inc., *London*
Prentice-Hall of Australia Pty. Limited, *Sydney*
Prentice-Hall of Canada, Ltd., *Toronto*
Prentice-Hall of India Private Limited, *New Delhi*
Prentice-Hall of Japan, Inc., *Tokyo*
Prentice-Hall of Southeast Asia Pte. Ltd., *Singapore*
Whitehall Books Limited, *Wellington, New Zealand*

*Without the Encouragement, Patience, Love, and Substantive Content Contributions From My Wife, This Book Could Never Have Been Written. I Dedicate This Book to Marilyn.*

# 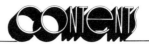 CONTENTS

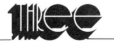

## Assessment of hearing handicap: self-report procedures   49

## Aural rehabilitation: an orientation   78

## Aural rehabilitation groups: a sample program   106

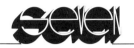

## Special populations

## Appendix   *141*

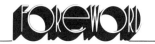

With the information explosion of recent years there has been a proliferation of knowledge in the areas of scientific and social inquiry. The speciality of communicative disorders has been no exception. While two decades ago a single textbook or "handbook" might have sufficed to provide the aspiring or practicing clinician with enlightenment on an array of communication handicaps, this is no longer possible—hence the decision to prepare a series of single-author texts.

As the title implies, the emphasis of this series, *Remediation of Communication Disorders,* is on therapy and treatment. The authors of each book were asked to provide information relative to anatomical and physiological aspects of each disorder, as well as pathology, etiology and diagnosis to the extent that an understanding of these factors bears on management procedures. In such relatively short books this was quite a challenge: to offer guidance without writing a "cookbook"; to be selective without being parochial; to offer theory without losing sight of practice. To this challenge the series' authors have risen magnificently.

The handicapping effects of hearing impairment have always been a primary professional interest of Thomas Giolas. The majority of his research efforts have centered around the assessment and prediction of the effects that loss of hearing have upon everyday life situations. What evolved was the certainty that implications for aural rehabilitation are more meaningful if the assessment of handicap is carefully carried out. In this book, Dr. Giolas ties together, in one volume, his clinical and research experience with the Hearing Performance Inventory, which he and his colleagues developed. Teachers and clinicians following the tenets of this book, rather than drill-like forms of therapy will likely find that their adult hearing-impaired patients are better served.

FREDERICK N. MARTIN
Series Editor

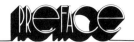
PREFACE

This book is concerned with the handicapping effect of hearing impairment and *aural rehabilitation.* It attempts to acquaint the reader with what it means to have a hearing impairment of sufficient severity to interfere with functional communication. The focus is on persons who have acquired a hearing impairment in adulthood and the unique communication and adjustment problems which may develop. A systematic differentiation is made between *hearing impairment* and *hearing handicap.* Hearing impairment is used as a generic term referring to any organic hearing problem regardless of etiology or degree. Hearing handicap is used to refer to the ways the hearing impairment has affected a person's everyday life situation. The overall goal of this book is to encourage audiology to move beyond the evaluation of hearing impairment and concentrate as much, if not more, on the assessment and management of hearing handicap. Accordingly, this book concentrates on the rehabilitative activities designed to assist hearing-impaired persons achieve their optimal potential in communication. Auditory and nonauditory procedures for assessing hearing handicap are discussed in detail. A Comprehensive Aural Rehabilitation Program is developed, followed by a sample eight-week program for working with a group of hearing-handicapped adults and their families. Specific modifications of these programs are suggested for persons with hearing impairments which are age-related, unilateral, or of sudden onset.

It is hoped that this book will serve as a stimulus to interest the reader in the rehabilitative needs of the adventitiously hearing-handicapped adult.

This book represents the strong influence of at least four colleagues who entered my life early in my career and remain close friends. Those who have read the works of Louise M. Ward, Elizabeth J. Webster, and Edwin W. Martin will recognize the source of the basic philosophy of client respect that underlies the approach presented in this book. For their contribution to my early professional and personal life I would like to take this opportunity to thank them. I would also like to acknowledge my teacher and friend, Aubrey Epstein. His unwavering faith and support provided me with the confidence to accept the academic challenge he gives to all his students.

Special thanks are extended to Lucy Tilton and Paul Simison for their help in typing and preparing the manuscript for publication.

And finally, gratitude goes to Panayota Noufrios for her early and continued love and support.

THOMAS G. GIOLAS

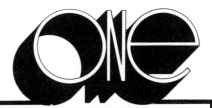

○ DEFINITION OF TERMS
○ TARGET POPULATION
○ THIS BOOK'S MISSION
○ PREREQUISITE INFORMATION
○ SUMMARY

# Introduction

Hearing plays an important and unique role in a person's developmental process. Initially in the early stages of life, infants respond to the world primarily in terms of how they feel physiologically and in terms of what is done to them physically in the course of their care. Hearing, through the infant's gross response to environmental sounds, serves to connect the infant with the physical environment beyond the confines of his or her own body. Shortly thereafter, the infant begins to respond more selectively and differentially to these environmental sounds, and this response lays the groundwork for the development of verbal communication skills. Verbal communication skills not only facilitate a smoother emotional, educational, and social growth process, but comprise the main component of the skills necessary for coping with the adult world. Shostrom (1967) believes that communication is the greatest problem two human beings face. Fleming (1972) describes communication as containing two basic elements: sending a message and receiving a message. People spend a great deal of their adult lives (1) attempting to make others understand what they are saying (sending a message) and (2) trying to understand (receive) what is being said to them.

The normal development of verbal communication skills depends to a great extent upon the ear's ability to receive and process acoustic energy, especially that which comprises the speech spectrum. Consequently, problems with the normal acquisition of language, speech, education, and vocational skills arise when hearing is impaired. For persons who have acquired hearing problems after they have reached adulthood, difficulties become acute in the areas of social interaction and performance in the employment setting, and often considerable strain is placed on interpersonal relationships.

The nature and severity of these problems depend on a number of factors. Hearing impairment can take one direction or a combination of several directions, each contributing to separate and overlapping problems. The severity of the resulting problems depends on (1) the amount of auditory deprivation (hearing loss), (2) the location along the auditory pathway where the damage lies (site of lesion), and (3) the person's age when the damage occurred (onset of impairment). Later, such factors as (1) the person's acceptance of the hearing impairment, (2) promptness in seeking professional assistance, (3) family support, and (4) the person's general approach to problem solving become extremely important in determining the adjustment pattern of a person who has acquired a hearing impairment in adulthood. Knowledge of these factors and how they interact is necessary in order to better understand the hearing-handicapped person.

## ○ DEFINITION OF TERMS

A number of terms are used to describe or refer to persons who are experiencing hearing difficulty. These terms are often used interchangeably and may carry a rather general meaning. However, that is not the case in this book. Throughout this book a number of terms, such as *hearing impairment, hearing loss,* and *hearing handicap,* will be used in a very specific way and will mean something quite different from one another. For example, to many people the sentence "Does the hearing impairment have a sufficiently severe hearing loss to result in a hearing handicap?" would seem somewhat forced at best and confusing at worst. However, in this book each of these terms (and many others to be discussed as they appear in subsequent chapters) have very specific definitions.

*Hearing impairment* is used here as a generic term referring to any organic hearing problem regardless of etiology or degree. We will also use this term within the context of the Davis and Silverman (1978) definition: "a deviation or change for the worse in either structure or function, usually outside the range of normal." In other words, *hearing impairment* emerges as the term to be used when reference is being made to the condition of abnormal hearing and no additional information regarding the impairment is indicated.

*Hearing loss* is used whenever specific reference is being made to a hearing impairment which is of a particular intensity magnitude, such as a 40dB hearing loss. At times *hearing level* will be used interchangeably with *hearing loss.*

Finally, *hearing handicap* will refer to the effect of the hearing impairment on the person's everyday situation. More specifically, we will faithfully follow the Davis and Silverman (1978) definition of this term: "the disadvantages imposed by an impairment sufficient to affect one's personal efficiency in the activities of daily living."

Employing these definitions, the previously introduced sentence, "Does the hearing impairment have a sufficiently severe hearing loss to result in a hearing handicap?" may be translated to mean "Does the hearing problem (hearing impairment) of unspecified nature have a sufficient acoustic energy loss (hearing loss) to cause interference in everyday listening tasks (hearing handicap)?"

Such close adherence to the specific use of these terms will go a long way in orienting the reader to the basic mission of this book: that is, to create an interest in the assessment of hearing handicap in adults and its treatment.

## ○ TARGET POPULATION

There are approximately 20 million children and adults in the United States who have hearing loss (Chalfant and Scheffelin 1969). In this society, one of the natural consequences of aging is the gradual reduction of hearing sensitivity. Figures 1–1 and 1–2 show the overall trend with age for men and women. With the prospect of an ever-increasing number of adults with appreciable hearing impairment, it is essential for professionals to look at the diagnostic and rehabilitative needs of this group.

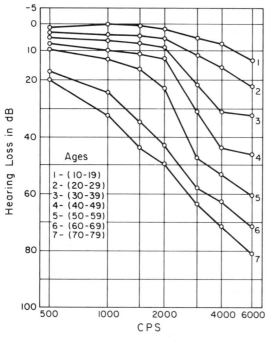

FIGURE 1–1 Median hearing losses of men in the total sample of the Wisconsin State Fair Survey. Data are referenced to ASA, 1951, audiometric zero, left ear only (A. Glorig et al., "1954 Wisconsin State Fair Hearing Survey," Monograph, American Academy of Otolaryngology—Head and Neck Surgery, 1957. Reprinted by permission.)

This book concentrates on the following target population:

1. Persons who have acquired a hearing impairment as adults.

2. Persons whose hearing impairment has resulted in partial or total loss of hearing, with gradual or sudden onset.

3. Persons whose hearing impairment has manifested itself in a hearing handicap.

4. Persons with either unilateral or bilateral hearing impairment.

Issues pertaining to congenitally deaf adults and children will be referred to as they facilitate the discussion of the adventitiously hearing-impaired adult.

4

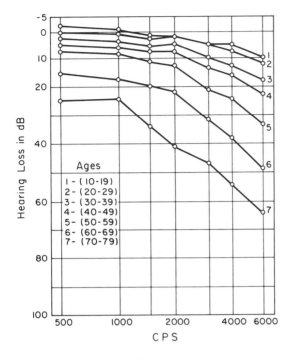

FIGURE 1–2 Median hearing losses for women in the total sample of the Wisconsin State Fair Survey. Data are referenced to ASA, 1951, audiometric zero. (From Glorig et al., 1957. Reproduced by permission.)

## ○ THIS BOOK'S MISSION

There is considerable interest on the part of professionals in the hearing-impaired child and in the diagnosis of hearing impairment in general. And rightly so. However, there is a greatly reduced interest in the rehabilitation of hearing-impaired adults who acquired their impairment as adults. These people are in dire need of rehabilitative procedures designed to asist them in coping with their medically irreversible hearing impairment. It is this group on which this book is focused. Chapters One and Two present the reader with basic and practical information about the handicapping effects of hearing impairment. These effects are discussed in terms of how the resulting communication problems affect the emotional, social, and occupational dimensions of the lives of persons with hearing impairments. It is concluded that rehabilitative programs designed to help persons cope with their hearing impairments are not only desirable but essential if these people are to continue living productive lives. Chapters Three and Four deal with the assessment of hearing handicap. Chapter Three describes the advantages and disadvantages of audiometric procedures as indicators of communication problems resulting from hearing impairment. Audiologists are encouraged to expand their view of these procedures and to incorporate them into their rehabilitative activities. Chapter Four reviews self-report procedures for assessing hearing handicap and develops a rationale for their use in overcoming some of the inadequacies of psychophysical measures.

Both chapters stress the need for assessment procedures which yield direct information regarding rehabilitative programs. Chapters Five, Six, and Seven focus on the nature of these programs. Chapter Five presents an orientation to the rehabilitation process, with an emphasis on the group discussion format. Chapter Six outlines a sample eight-week rehabilitation program. Chapter Seven addresses some of the modifications necessary for several special populations.

The book's mission can be summarized as follows:

1. To create an awareness of the rehabilitative needs of the hearing-impaired adult.
2. To provide detailed information necessary to design and conduct programs which will assist adults in learning to cope with their hearing impairments.

## ○ PREREQUISITE INFORMATION

It is assumed that the reader has a basic background in audiology and is knowledgeable in the areas of (1) elementary physics of sound, (2) anatomy and physiology of the ear, (3) basic ear pathology and treatment, and (4) standard pure tone and speech audiometric procedures. Reference to each of these areas will be made a number of times, but only in terms of the assessment and management of hearing handicap.

It is also assumed that the reader has a genuine interest in working with persons who have medically irreversible hearing impairments.

The primary purpose of the book is to create an awareness of the rehabilitative needs of the hearing-impaired adult. Persons acquiring a hearing impairment in adult-hood experience varying degrees of communication problems which adversely affect their social, occupational, and emotional lives. These problems are a function of the age at which the hearing impairment occurs, as well as the extent and physiological basis. Rehabilitation programs designed to help persons cope with their hearing impairment are not only desirable, but essential if these people are to continue to live productive lives.

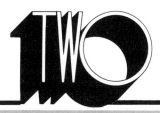

# What it means to have a hearing impairment

A hearing impairment that is acquired either gradually or precipitously and is extensive enough to interfere with the normal communication process creates a myriad of problems so complex that coping with the predominatly hearing world becomes quite difficult for hearing-impaired persons. The resulting adjustment problems can be numerous and severe. Prior to the onset of the hearing impairment, these persons were able to rely on their hearing to assist them in conducting the majority of their personal, social, and business affairs. They had been accustomed to functioning in a hearing world where people spoke to them; they heard and understood what was said, and all was well. Suddenly (or gradually) it has become apparent that they cannot depend completely on their hearing to function in these communication situations. The number of times they have misinterpreted what was said and have responded inappropriately has increased, and they have come to realize that they may need a new approach to handling their everyday affairs. In other words, the hearing-impaired person's typical mode of communication no longer works. This realization is quite disturbing, to say the least, and acceptance of it is quite an adjustment. Noble (1978) writes:

> The acquisition of partial deafness in adulthood can be particularly traumatic for an individual in an otherwise hearing social network. No preparation has been made for such a transition, and the solitary nature of the occurrence leaves the individual with a feeling of bereavement. Heaton (1968) has made a similar observation in regard to sighted people who become increasingly blind. Even in a sympathetic social environment, the person who, through disease or injury, sustains a hearing loss is largely alone in this partially deaf world.(p. 18)

What form do these adjustment patterns take? There is no question in most clinicians' minds that they differ from person to person regardless of the nature of the hearing impairment. The form is most likely dependent on how the person typically handles most serious problems in life.

○ PERSONAL ADJUSTMENT PATTERNS

Rousey (1971) writes that the nature of the adjustment pattern one uses is closely related to the way common human emotions known as affects are inappropriately expressed as a result of a threat to one's well-being and personal integrity. *Affects* are defined as feelings of love, longing, jealousy, mortification, pain, and mourning at one end of the continuum of feeling, and as feelings of hatred, anger, and rage at the opposite pole. Rousey (1971) views hearing impairment as constituting a sufficient threat to " . . . exacerbate long-standing problems in dealing with affect." In other words, the hearing impairment is seen as a sufficiently serious irritant to trigger off a number of behaviors typically used to deal with severe frustration and personal threat.

Hearing-impaired persons must then rely on pre-hearing-impairment internal affects to respond to their environment. If these internal affects are relatively healthy they will serve them well. However, if they are unstable, the result may be the opposite.

According to Rousey (1971), the major reactions associated with hearing impairment are (1) projection and (2) denial. As defined by Rousey, *projection* is what occurs when "an individual attributes to others in his environment some unpleasant wishes and feelings that he is experiencing within himself" (p. 387).

*Denial* is defined by Rousey (1971) as defensive behavior used when one is under severe attack by internal stress or external pressures and in situations where affects are threatening to become uncontrollable. Evidences of the defense mechanism of denial are seen daily in the audiology clinic. There are those who refuse to acknowledge that they need a hearing aid when it's quite clear to the audiologist as well as to the family. More seriously, there's the deaf child's parent who refuses to accept the diagnosis of hearing impairment and will spend many more months and even years looking for a more favorable diagnosis, wasting precious habilitative years.

Once the defense mechanisms are terminated or let down temporarily (or even while they are being used), the hearing-impaired person may experience one or more affect. Rousey (1971) states that two affects typically associated with hearing impairment are *mourning* and *mortification*. Each of these reactions have been observed by this author in one form or another in hearing-impaired persons.

One patient who acquired a sudden severe hearing loss in both ears actually spoke of the "death" of her hearing. And for a period she went through a mourning experience. A second person displayed the affect of mortification in the form of shame. He was convinced that he would be ostracized or even punished for having a hearing impairment. Rousey (1971) writes that these feelings are often considered derivatives of shame. Still another woman displayed mortification in a more general sense by devoting an inordinate amount of time to wondering why such an awful thing could happen to her.

One of the more observable reactions to a loss of hearing of differing degrees is the constant struggle with feelings of *depression*. The depression varies from person to person, even from day to day, and is often not readily explainable in terms of the degree to which the hearing loss has interfered with verbal communication. Ramsdell (1978) attempts to explain these feelings of depression as a function of the way the hearing impairment has interfered with three levels of hearing: (1) the symbolic, (2) the signal or warning, and (3) the primitive. While interference with all three of these hearing levels contributes in varying degrees to the depression, interference with the primitive level is often viewed as contributing the most.

The *primitive level* of hearing is the way normally hearing people add depth to the world around them. Even though they are mostly unaware of it, they are constantly extending their environment beyond the person with whom they are speaking and even beyond their sphere of vision by attending to background sounds (noises in other rooms, etc.) that are peculiar to that particular environment. For example, consider the person who is in a lecture hall listening to a speaker. In addition to this conscious, deliberate use of hearing, the person is also attending in a somewhat semiconscious way to a number of environmental background sounds such as those made by an air conditioner or by people who are shuffling or coughing randomly. All these background sounds contribute to making the total environment more alive and acoustically multidimensional. They connect the normally hearing person with the world much more fully than the conscious, deliberate level of hearing does by itself.

When a hearing impairment becomes sufficiently extensive to interfere with or diminish the hearing of the auditory background of daily living, confusion and depression often occur, and the hearing-impaired person may experience the world as dead. One person who had acquired a sudden severe bilateral hearing loss reported that the sudden silence gave her the feeling that something ominous had happened in the world and that everyone was mourning a death. Ramsdell (1978) discusses the role of the primitive level of hearing as follows:

> It relates us to the world at a very primitive level, somewhere below the level of clear consciousness and perception. The loss of this feeling or relationship with the world is the major cause of the well-recognized feeling of "deadness" and also of the depression that permeates the suddenly deafened and, to a lesser degree, those in whom deafness develops gradually. (p. 501)

As changes in the environmental sounds occur and are responded to, a new phenomenon emerges. The normally hearing person is no longer only hearing these sounds on the primitive level, but has moved on to a more conscious level of hearing. In the example used earlier, the person listening on a semiconscious level (the primitive level) to the air conditioner uses that sound as one parameter to define the environment, and when the air conditioner stops because the room has reached the desired temperature, the person quickly notices that the room acoustics have changed and are now minus that sound. If one multiplies that event by a number of such changes in auditory events occurring in one's auditory world, one can begin to see that normal hearing provides the feeling that the room is not only alive but ever changing. It is this phenomenon of a changing world that provides the person with a sense of security and a readiness for immediate changes. For many hearing-impaired persons, the loss of the auditory cues that indicate these changes is particularly annoying, especially because they do not quite understand what has taken place.

In summary, the primitive level of hearing provides a very important and basic contribution to a person's general feeling of security. It is the basic ingredient which creates a background of feeling, which Ramsdell (1978) calls an affective tone (p. 501). In its semiconscious listening stage it connects people with their immediate auditory environment, helping them to feel a part of a living, active world. As they become aware of the auditory background of daily living, they are alerted to changes occurring and are in a state of readiness to react appropriately. Interference with this level of hearing causes a number of problems, which will be discussed in Chapter Five along with ways to assist the hearing-impaired person in coping with these problems. Rehabilitation of persons experiencing sudden severe hearing impairments, as well of as those experiencing gradual hearing impairments, will be discussed.

The second level of hearing, which Ramsdell (1978) calls the *signal level* or *warning level*, consists of a more conscious level of listening which provides people with valuable information about what's going on in the world around them. Normally hearing persons are constantly aware of sounds within their hearing range. For example, they are often aware of what's going on in other rooms of the house, whether someone is walking around upstairs or coming down the stairs, when someone comes into the room (even if that person is out of their line of vision), from which direction a sound is coming, whether someone in another car is blowing a horn at them, and a host of other auditory events. These signals serve as warnings and allow normally hearing persons to react appropriately. When they hear the siren of an ambulance or police car, they typically slow down and pull to the right shoulder of the road. Failure to do so can certainly be embarrassing if not downright dangerous. The security afforded normally hearing persons as a result of their ability to hear most sounds within their range of hearing as well as their ability to identify from which direction a sound is coming must not be underestimated.

The highest and most refined level of hearing is that level which allows people to organize auditory events around them into meaningful language units or symbols. These symbols are used to communicate verbally with others. Ramsdell (1978) calls this level the *symbolic level*. The symbolic level requires the best hearing acuity of the three levels described so far, and interference with this level causes a host of communication problems. These problems and the conditions under which they occur will be the topic of the next section.

## ○ COMMUNICATION PROBLEMS

The primary consequence of a hearing impairment is the possible loss of verbal communication efficiency. For persons who have heard normally all their lives, the auditory mode has played the primary role in the acquisition and execution of verbal communication. While there is no question that nonverbal cues such as facial expressions, lip movements, body positions, and gestures add much to the nuances of meanings, persons who grew up with normal hearing depend on that hearing to receive the major portion of the verbal message.

In the previous section we discussed some of the psychological implications associated with adjusting to an interruption of the verbal communication process. This section will describe some of the common communication problems experienced by adults who have acquired hearing impairments.

The communication problems typically associated with persons who acquired hearing impairments in adulthood result from (1) a breakdown or a degree of deterioration of the auditory processing mechanism and (2) the effect of the organic condition (hearing impairment) on the reception and interpretation of the speech code. A discussion of the physiological status of the damaged auditory mechanism is not appropriate here. It is assumed that the reader has this basic understanding of how the ear functions. For a quick review of the subject, the reader may refer to excellent discussions in Davis and Silverman (1978). The major focus of this discussion is on the effect of the organic condition on the communication problems associated with the given hearing impairment.

In discussing the communication problems associated with hearing impairment, our concerns are threefold: (1) the effect of loss of intensity, (2) the effect of loss of speech discrimination ability, and (3) the contribution of environmental conditions to overall communication effectiveness. Each of these conditions will be discussed separately. The reader is reminded that the material is being presented here in a overview; the purpose is to give the reader a feel for the handicapping effects of a hearing impairment. Conditions which lend themselves to remediation will be covered in more depth in Chapters Five and Seven.

### intensity of the signal

One of the common results of a hearing impairment is that speech and other auditory signals are not processed by the impaired auditory mechanism at normal intensity levels. As a result, functioning in normal everyday listening situations is rendered more difficult from the standpoint of *hearing* and *understanding* what is being said.[1] For example, it is generally accepted that conversational speech is heard at approximately 45 dB HL. A person who has an audiometrically measured hearing level of 45 dB (ANSI) would be receiving normal conversational speech quite faintly, missing faint speech altogether, and receiving loud speech at a comfortable level. The preceding example represents listening in a quiet setting. Typical noisy settings would create an even more difficult listening task for the hearing-impaired person. Such listening conditions would cause the person considerable difficulty in many talking, learning, and working situations.

The problem is further complicated when one recognizes that acoustic speech covers a wide range of intensity. Individual speech phonemes vary, depending on how they are measured, as much as 30 to 35 dB, with the fricative ($\theta$) representing the phoneme containing the lowest overall intensity and the vowel ( ) containing the highest overall intensity. This is further complicated by the fact that conversational speech is a dynamic process altering the intensity range of the message from moment to moment depending on the talker's speaking volume, stress patterns, and distance from the listener.

Boothroyd (1978) addresses the effect of this dynamic range on the listener. He writes:

> If, for example, the speech signal is lowered in intensity until the weak fricative [$\theta$] becomes unidentifiable, a further reduction of approximately 30 dB is needed before the strong vowel [ɔ] becomes unidentifiable (Fletcher 1953, Chapter Four). Similarly, if a white noise masking signal is increased in intensity until it begins to affect phoneme recognition, another 30 dB increase is necessary before phoneme recognition approaches zero (Miller 1947). And in filtering experiments carried out by French and Steinberg (1947), it has been found that there is a difference of roughly 30 dB between the intensity at which a frequency band begins to contribute to phoneme recognition and the intensity at which its contribution reaches a maximum. (p. 118)

The point of this discussion is to say the obvious. First, that speech must be loud enough to be useful to the listener; second, that hearing impairment frequently reduces the intensity of speech. The degree and nature of the alteration of speech with respect to intensity are functions of an interaction between (1) the acoustic parameters of individual phonemes, (2) the conversational context (prosodic features) in which they are being produced, and (3) the hearing impairment of the listener. The handicapping effect and its measurement and rehabilitation are the subjects of subsequent chapters.

[1]For purposes of this discussion, *hearing* is defined as being aware of an auditory signal, and *understanding* is defined as hearing the words the other person is saying clearly enough to be able to participate in the conversation.

### speech discrimination

One of the more common problems of persons with hearing impairments is the clarity of the speech to which they are listening. Depending on the nature of the impairment, speech will be distorted to some degree. Audiologists are often told: "Speech is loud enough for me; it's just not clear enough"; or "Now that I'm wearing my hearing aid, I can hear people; I just can't understand what they are saying." Audiologists refer to this condition as a problem in *speech discrimination*. The process of measuring speech discrimination for rehabilitative purposes will be discussed in Chapter Three.

For the purposes of this discussion, it is sufficient to state that speech discrimination is generally measured by presenting hearing-impaired persons with a speech message at a comfortable listening level and obtaining a measure of how well they were able to repeat what was said. It is assumed that there is a close relationship between the ability to repeat the speech message presented and the level of difficulty that is experienced in most conversational situations. While there are certainly a number of other factors contributing to a person's communicative efficiency, the degree to which the speech signal is received clearly plays a major role. Therefore, we must discuss speech discrimination as a function of hearing impairment so that we may better understand its handicapping effect. Furthermore, knowledge of the kind of speech errors made by a given individual will have rehabilitative value.

A number of studies have been conducted dealing with the adult's ability to identify various components of the speech signal under a number of acoustic conditions. Most of these studies were conducted using persons with normal hearing who listened to experimentally degraded messages. In many cases the results of these studies have direct application to hearing-impaired adults. This is especially so for the population of major concern in this book: those adults who have grown up hearing normally, who have had the benefit of acoustic, linguistic, and environmental redundancy and who then find themselves in a position where this redundancy is slowly (or suddenly) diminishing. Owens and his colleagues have conducted a number of studies (1968a, 1968b, 1972, 1974) using hearing-impaired persons and looking at their vowel and consonant discrimination ability. It seems appropriate to center the discussion of speech discrimination problems around the Owens studies, bringing in other research findings where applicable.

The purpose of this discussion is to look at the kinds of vowel and consonant errors made by persons with hearing impairment in order to obtain some insight into their speech discrimination difficulties. In later sections of this chapter we will discuss other factors influencing the overall problem of understanding connected speech in an everyday listening situation.

14

*Vowel Discrimination.*   What does the spoken message sound like to hearing-impaired persons? Which speech categories are interfered with as a result of their auditory configuration and which categories are more available to them? It was generally accepted that persons with acquired hearing impairments experienced less difficulty identifying vowels than consonants regardless of their audiometric configuration. However, investigators such as Schultz (1964) and Oyer and Dounda (1959) suggested that vowel discrimination is not a simple function and that it is likely that persons with different pathologies perceive vowels differently. Owens, Talbott, and Schubert (1968b) set out to look at the discrimination performance of hearing-impaired persons. A series of 288 multiple choice items was developed to test all common vowels and diphthongs. The results indicated that when test items of this nature were presented to hearing-impaired persons whose speech discrimination scores ranged from 20% to 70% with a mean of 46.0% using the CID W-22 word series, a surprisingly low number of vowel errors were made ($\overline{X}$ of 93.6%), suggesting that the decreased discrimination scores obtained on the W-22 word lists were more a function of consonant errors than vowel errors. Furthermore, when the subjects were divided into etiology groups (Menières, noise-induced, presbycusis, and other sensorineural) no differences emerged between the subgroups. The Shultz (1964) and Oyer and Dounda (1959) suggestions were not supported. It is clear that the major contributor to the speech discrimination problem experienced by hearing-impaired adults is their failure to perceive the consonant phonemes as clearly as they once did.

It is important to note that this writer does not intend to suggest that there is not consonant influence and even spillover energy present in the vowels that are perceived, whether they are heard normally as a result of good hearing in the lower audiometric frequencies or amplified through a hearing aid. On the contrary, the reverse is true; it is only because the adjacent consonants alter the enclosed vowels that hearing-impaired persons are able to function as well as they do in most listening situations. This phenomenon is referred to as the coarticulation effect of adjacent speech sounds. Gay (1970) studied the influence of vowel environment on consonant identification under different filtering conditions. Vowels were found to be highly intelligible under almost all conditions, while consonant-vowel combinations showed a great deal of resistance to the filtering effects. The role of coarticulation, transients, and other acoustic critical features has been studied extensively by Liberman, Cooper, Shankweiler, and Studdert-Kennedy (1967). Cole and Scott (1974), Gay (1970), and others clearly show that perception of speech is linked to a set of multiple cues in the speech spectrum that interact simultaneously to result in the identification of speech sounds.

*Consonant Discrimination.* It is generally accepted that persons with high-frequency hearing losses will yield decreased speech discrimination scores when tested using one of several monosyllabic word lists. It is further suggested that the greater the hearing loss in the high frequencies, the poorer the discrimination score. We have learned in the previous section that this decreased speech discrimination ability is not primarily a function of vowel discrimination, but probably more a function of poor consonant discrimination. This assumption is supported time and time again by a number of studies using normal listeners (Miller and Nicely 1955). In a series of three studies (1968, 1972, 1974) Owens and his colleagues attempted to describe the consonant discrimination performance of hearing-impaired persons by using persons with a number of specific audiometric configurations and medical etiologies. A discussion of these studies will provide the reader with a picture of which consonant phonemes the hearing-impaired person does not identify and which ones the person assumes he or she has heard.

Owens and Schubert (1968a) investigated the consonant errors made by hearing-impaired persons on speech discrimination test lists employing a closed set. These lists were specifically designed to assess most of the voiced and unvoiced consonants in both the initial and final positions. The subjects were English-speaking adults with hearing impairments who scored in range from 20% to 70% on a W-22 list. Etiology of hearing impairment did not enter into the selection. The following results are of interest here:

1. Confusion between unvoiced and voiced consonants rarely occurred.

2. The (r) and (l) were rarely confused with other phonemes, and nasals were seldom confused with other phonemes.

3. Table 2–1 contains a list of consonants missed in terms of probabilities for initial and final positions. The probability of error was highest for the (p) and lowest for the (g) in the initial position, and the probability of error was highest for the (k) and lowest for the (v) in the final position. The probability of error for most phonemes tended to be higher when they were tested in the final as opposed to the initial positions. The listeners experienced inordinate difficulty in discriminating between (f-$\theta$) and (v-ð) when both phonemes were among the response foils and one pair was the stimulus.

4. Table 2–2 summarizes an analysis that was made of the error responses in order to determine the phonemes most often substituted for the various stimulus phonemes. As can be seen, discrimination difficulty was related to both position and manner of articulation.

A second study was conducted by Owens, Benedict, and Schubert (1972) in order to allow for a closer look at consonant phonemic errors as a function of more rigidly defined audiometric configurations and kinds of hearing impairment. A revised version of the Owens and Schubert (1968a) series of multiple choice items was used, and the subjects had the following pure tone configurations: (1) flat thresholds within 10 dB of a best-fitting

TABLE 2–1
Probability of Error on Phonemes Tested
in the Initial and Final Positions

| STIMULUS | PROBABILITY OF ERROR | |
|---|---|---|
| PHONEMES | INITIAL | FINAL |
| /p/ | 0.43 | 0.55 |
| /dʒ/ | 0.26 | 0.52 |
| /v/ | 0.11 | 0.48 |
| /s/ | 0.39 | 0.48 |
| /t/ | 0.35 | 0.45 |
| /k/ | 0.45 | 0.45 |
| /b/ | 0.33 | 0.38 |
| /f/ | 0.17 | 0.35 |
| /t/ | 0.29 | 0.35 |
| /d/ | 0.30 | 9.33 |
| /θ/ | 0.33 | 0.32 |
| /z/ | — | 0.27 |
| /ʃ/ | 0.33 | 0.23 |
| /g/ | 0.16 | 0.22 |
| /ʒ/ | 0.45 | — |
| /h/ | 0.23 | — |
| /w/ | 0.18 | — |
| /l/ | 0.08 | 0.05 |
| /r/ | 0.06 | 0.05 |
| /j/ | 0.08 | — |
| /m/ | — | 0.05 |
| /n/ | — | 0.03 |

E. Owens and E. D. Schubert, "The Development of Consonant Items for
Speech Discrimination Testing," *Journal of Speech and Hearing Research*,
11 (1968), pp. 656–667. Reprinted by permission.

horizontal line, from 500 Hz to 8000 Hz (16 subjects); (2) mild slope with
a consistent downward slope from 500 Hz to 4000Hz, not greater than 15
dB and not less than 10 dB per octave (18 subjects); and (3) sharp slope,
with consistent downward slope of 20 dB or more per octave from 500 Hz
to 4000 Hz (14 subjects). A group of 27 subjects with normal hearing were
also included in the 1972 study, but this will be discussed in a later section.
Several interesting findings were obtained. Scores on the Owens and Schubert (1968a) test items were consistently poorer than on the W-22 list, both
overall and for each subgroup. The (s), (ʃ), (tʃ), (d ʒ) and the initial (t) and
( ) were easily identified by patients with flat pure tone configurations but
were difficult for patients with sharp falling slopes from 500 Hz to 4000 Hz.
Owens, Benedict, and Schubert (1972) write:

> Marked differences in identifiability are seen for the /s, ʃ, tʃ, dʒ/ in both
> the final and initial positions, and for the /t/ and /θ/ in the initial position
> only. For these phonemes the probability of error increases consistently
> with the steepness of the high-tone slope. The only other differences that

## TABLE 2-2
### Phonemes Likely to Be Substituted for the Stimulus Phonemes

Numbers in the table are probabilities obtained by dividing the number of times a particular phoneme was substituted for the stimulus, by the number of chances (trials) for such substitutions. Probabilities less than 0.10 were omitted. The upper number in each cell represents substitutions in the initial position; the bottom number, substitutions in the final position.

**RESPONSES**

**(a) Unvoiced Stimulus Phonemes**

| | /p/ | /t/ | /k/ | /t/ | /s/ | /ʃ/ | /f/ | /θ/ | /h/ |
|---|---|---|---|---|---|---|---|---|---|
| /p/ | — | 0.24 / 0.32 | 0.15 / 0.18 | — | — | — | 0.11 / 0.21 | 0.18 / 0.10 | — |
| /t/ | 0.21 / 0.17 | — | 0.11 / 0.17 | — | — | — | — / 0.10 | 0.10 / 0.12 | — |
| /k/ | 0.16 / 0.15 | — | 0.32 / 0.31 | — | — | — | — | — | — |
| /t/ | — / 0.16 | 0.11 / 0.22 | 0.11 / 0.11 | — | — | 0.11 | — | 0.16 / 0.23 | — |
| /s/ | — / 0.14 | — / 0.19 | — | 0.10 | — | — | 0.32 / 0.26 | 0.29 / 0.46 | — |
| /ʃ/ | — | — | — | 0.16 | 0.17 / 0.14 | — | — | 0.16 | — |
| /f/ | — / 0.14 | — / 0.15 | 0.11 | — | 0.11 / 0.12 | — | — | — | — |
| /e/ | — / 0.30 | — / 0.15 | — | — | 0.19 | — | — | — | — |
| /h/ | 0.13 | — | — | — | — | — | 0.13 | — | — |

**(b) Voiced**

| | /b/ | /d/ | /g/ | /dʒ/ | /z/ | /v/ | /ð/ | /r/ | /l/ | /w/ | /j/ |
|---|---|---|---|---|---|---|---|---|---|---|---|
| /b/ | — | 0.16 / 0.21 | — | — | — | 0.32 / 0.18 | *0.60 | — | 0.10 | — | — |
| /d/ | 0.18 / 0.14 | — | 0.15 / 0.15 | — | *0.15 / 0.11 | — / 0.14 | *0.25 | — | — | — | — |
| /g/ | — | 0.15 | — | — / 0.11 | — / 0.10 | — | — | — | — | — | — |
| /dʒ/ | *0.30 | 0.31 | 0.18 | — | — / 0.14 | 0.10 / 0.11 | — | 0.10 | — | — | 0.10 |
| /z/ | — | *0.10 | — | — | — | *0.50 / 0.23 | — | — | — | — | — |
| /v/ | — / 0.10 | — / 0.26 | — | — | *0.10 / 0.20 | — | — | — | — | — | — |
| /ð/ | *0.25 | — | — | — | — | — | — | 0.15 | — | — | — |
| /r/ | — | — | — | — | — | — | — | — | — | — | — |
| /l/ | — | — | — | — | — | — | — | 0.25 | — | — | — |
| /w/ | — | — | — | — | — | — | — | — | — | — | — |
| /j/ | — | — | — | — | — | *0.15 | — | — | — | — | — |

*Trials = 20 (one item for 20 patients). Other trials = 40 or more.

E. Owens and E. D. Schubert, "The Development of Consonant Items for Speech Discrimination Testing," *Journal of Speech and Hearing Research*, 11 (1968), pp. 656–667. Reprinted by permission.

appear worthy of note are for the final /b/ and /d/, which show relatively higher error probabilities for the flat configurations, but no consistent trends for the other three configuration groups. (p. 313)

The identification of the (s) and the initial (t) and (θ) was highly dependent upon energy in the frequency range above 2000 Hz, whereas identification of the ( ʃ, tʃ, dʒ) was highly dependent upon the range between 1000 Hz and 2000 Hz. The (b) and (d) were more difficult with flat configuration. Figure 2–1 illustrates the phonemic errors made as a function of pure tone configuration.

In general, the phonemes missed were similar to those presented in the Owens and Schubert (1968a) study, and only a few of the stimulus phonemes appear to be related to pure tone configuration. Owens, Benedict, and Schubert (1972) write:

> Thus, for the phonemes and pure-tone configurations studied here, only a few of the stimulus phonemes appear to be related in specific ways to the configurations. Patients with flat configurations, 500 to 8000 Hz, seemingly regardless of threshold level and overall score, experienced relatively little difficulty in identifying /s/, / ʃ /, / tʃ /, /dʒ/, initial /t/, and intitial / θ /. Patients with flat configurations to 2000 Hz and a sharp cut-off thereafter experienced difficulty in identifying /s/, initial /t/, and initial / θ /, but little difficulty in identifying / ʃ /, / tʃ /, and /dʒ/. For the remaining patients, no specific relations appeared between pure-tone configurations and the identification of particular phonemes. (pp. 316-317)

Finally, phonemic substitutions were not related to a particular pure tone configuration. These findings were supported by a third study that was conducted by Owens and Sher (1974).

In summary, with regard to vowel and consonant discrimination it may be concluded that: (1) Persons with hearing impairments that have been corrected by amplification do not have serious discrimination problems with vowels; (2) such persons experience varying degrees of difficulty with consonants, depending upon the audiometric configuration; (3) there is no systematic set of error responses associated with etiology; and (4) normally hearing persons listening to distorted speech produce error responses quite similar to those of hearing-impaired persons. This last finding is most helpful to the clinician who wishes to generalize from data obtained with normally hearing persons and apply it to hearing-impaired persons. Probably the most important clinical implication of these results is the consistent finding that hearing above 2000 Hz plays an extremely important role in speech discrimination. A thorough study of the Owens research discussed here is strongly recommended and will prove enlightening and clinically helpful.

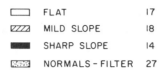

FLAT            17
MILD SLOPE      18
SHARP SLOPE     14
NORMALS – FILTER  27

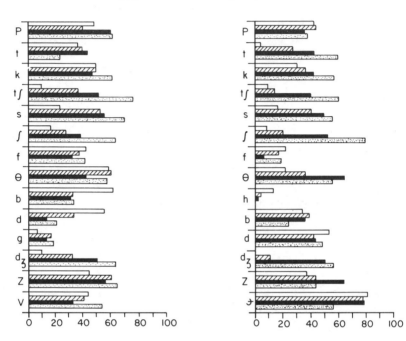

PROBABILITY OF ERROR

FIGURE 2–1 Probability of Error on Individual Phonemes (Final Position) for Subjects with Certain Pure-Tone Configurations and Probability of Error on Individual Phonemes (Initial Position) for Subjects with Certain Pure-Tone Configurations. (E. Owens and N. Benedict, "Consonant Phonemic Errors Associated with Pure-Tone Configurations and Certain Kinds of Hearing Aid Impairment," *Journal of Speech and Hearing Research,* 15 (1972), pp. 308–322. Reprinted by permission.)

### environmental conditions

***Noise Environment.*** One of the most common complaints expressed by persons with sensorineural hearing impairments is that they have the most difficulty understanding speech when the listening condition contains background noise. Typical noisy conditions include:

1. Background music in restaurants, music from hi-fi sets in the home, music superimposed on tv sound tracks.
2. Noises produced by household machinery such as air conditioners, dehumidifiers, dishwashers, window fans.

TABLE 2–3
Approximate Sound-Pressure Levels of
Familiar Environmental Sounds

DECIBELS

| | | |
|---|---|---|
| Jet engine (100 feet) | 140 | Pain threshold |
| | — | Air raid siren |
| Riveting gun | 130 | Threshold of feeling (tickle) |
| | — | |
| Thunder clap | 120 | Turbine generators |
| Modern discotheque | — | |
| | 110 | Loud shout (1 foot) |
| Power lawnmower | — | Diesel truck (high speed) |
| N.Y. subway | 100 | Motorcycle (no muffler) |
| Jackhammer | — | Electric blender |
| Shouted speech | 90 | Speech interference level |
| | — | City traffic (inside car) |
| | 80 | Loud singing (not amplified) |
| | — | |
| Noisy restaurant | 70 | |
| | — | |
| | 60 | Normal speaking level |
| | — | |
| | 50 | Average office |
| Quiet residence | — | |
| | 40 | Quiet office |
| | — | |
| | 30 | Faint whisper |

D. M. Lipscomb, "Noise in the Environment: The Problem." Maco Audiological
Library Series, VIII (1970), Report No. 1, pp. 1–6.

3. The overall noise produced by numbers of people talking simultaneously such as in a party setting.

Table 2–3 lists a number of familiar environmental noises and their dB levels. If you keep in mind that normal conversational speech occurs at approximately 77 dB SPL, it becomes apparent that if many of these sounds occur in the background while conversation is attempted, much of the speech message will be rendered unintelligible even if hearing is normal.

It must be pointed out that whatever the original physical characteristics of a sound (speech, background music, etc.), when it is introduced into a particular room it is altered considerably by the particular acoustic characteristics of that room. At times these changes, including the intensity ratio between the primary source (speech) and various background sounds, combine to render conversational speech difficult to understand even for persons with normal hearing. More importantly, there is considerable evidence that persons with sensorineural hearing impairments experience considerably more difficulty understanding speech than do persons with normal hearing when listening to speech under identical conditions (Tillman, Carhart, and Olsen 1974; Nabelek and Pickett 1974a, 1974b; Crum and Tillman 1973). The hearing impairment produces limited intensity as well as frequency and temporal characteristics which require more favorable room acoustics for adequate speech intelligibility.

This differential effect is a function of the interaction of a number of acoustic parameters such as (1) the intensity ratio between the speaker's voice and the ambient noise level, (2) the reverberation characteristics of the room and the resultant reverberation time, and (3) whether or not the precedence effect is operating (Ross 1978). These factors, coupled with an individual's particular audiometric configuration, can be disastrous to the ability to understand conversational speech.

A full discussion of these phenomenon is beyond the scope of this book. For a more complete understanding of the deleterious effects of poor room acoustics, the reader may consult Ross (1978).

The impact of personal amplification (hearing aids) on speech intelligibility for the hearing-impaired person will be discussed in a later section. However, to complete the discussion of why hearing-impaired persons may experience difficulty in certain noise situations, it should be noted that in some cases amplification (1) creates an upward spread of masking phenomena that obscure the valuable high frequencies essential to good speech discrimination or (2) creates a tolerance problem that if not properly considered will produce unnecessary distortion.

Finally, it has been stated that persons with sensorineural hearing impairments experience varying degrees of difficulty understanding conversational speech in settings where there is background noise. The explanation given here has been that this phenomenon is the result of a combination of (1) ambient noise levels due to an interaction between primary signals, (2) the particular acoustics of the room, and (3) the nature of the individual's hearing impairment. With regard to the role played by room acoustics, Ross (1978) writes:

> The point of view has been expressed that it is the amplitude and time of arrival of these reflected sound patterns rather than reverberation time per se which determine intelligibility under reverberant conditions (Lochner and Burger 1964). The reverberation time and room volume "set the stage" while the sound reflections do the acting. These reflections of an ongoing speech signal are a particularly deceptive masking source. They are timelocked in an overlapping manner to the speech and they occur only when speech is being emitted. A room may appear to have good acoustic qualities because of a low ambient noise level, but this factor cannot predict the masking effect of reflected speech sounds.

***Communication Settings.*** We have been discussing sensorineural hearing impairment in terms of its effect on communication. So far we have considered the roles played by these conditions: (1) the physical characteristics of the environment (room acoustics); (2) the frequency, intensity, and time restriction of the spoken message (hearing impairment); (3) personal amplification (the hearing aid); and (4) the hearing-impaired person's adjustment to the hearing impairment. The interactions of these conditions with a number of other factors such as the history of the hearing impairment will be dealt with later on in this chapter.

In order to complete the picture, it is important to discuss a host of additonal conditions which are imposed by the communication setting itself and which have a great influence on the success or failure of a communication event. These conditions include (1) the nature and purpose of the conversation, (2) the number of persons involved in the conversation, and (3) the relationship of the speaker(s) to the hearing-impaired person. Consequently, in order to fully appreciate what it means to have a hearing impairment, the role of communication settings must be explored.

One of the most comprehensive studies exploring the social implications of hearing impairment was conducted at the University of Pittsburgh under the direction of Drs. Emily Nett, Leo Doerfler, and Jack Mathews (1960). The investigation was sponsored by the Vocational Rehabilitation Administration and was designed to study hard-of-hearing adults and the effect of hearing impairment on their daily life experiences. A total of 378 hearing-impaired persons were interviewed and tested both audiologically and psychologically. In addition, 246 spouses, friends, relatives, and work associates were interviewed. The critical incident interviewing technique (Flanagan 1954) was used with all subjects. While a number of findings emerged, it is the results of these interviews which assist us in gaining some insights into the communication problems experienced by the hearing-impaired adult.

A brief description of the critical incident interviewing technique is in order, because the discussion to follow will be in terms of respondents' critical incident reports. This technique is basically an "inductive method of building up generalizations by abstracting them from a large number of concrete events rather than by inferring them deductively from some super-ordinate concept of definition" (Flanagan 1954). In discussing the critical incident, Flanagan writes:

> By an incident is meant any observable human activity that is sufficiently complete in itself to permit inferences and predictions to be made about the person performing the act. To be critical, an incident must occur in a situation where the purpose or intent of the act seems fairly clear to the observer and where its consequences are sufficiently definite to leave little doubt concerning its effects. (p. 327)

In the University of Pittsburgh study, the following instructions were given to each interviewee:

I am conducting a study to find out how your hearing loss affects your daily life. In order to find out I would like you to tell me about times when you have had some difficulty because of your hearing loss. I will then ask you specific questions about each of these times so that I know exactly what happened. To answer these questions will require some thought, but I think you will be able to remember times of the kind I have in mind. Can you tell me how your hearing loss is affecting or has affected your life? (Nett, Doerfler, and Mathews 1960, p. 35)

More specific questions were then asked about each reported incident. These questions concerned the time, place, people involved, action taken, and feelings about the situation. Each interview was conducted by a research team which was familiar with Flanagan's interviewing technique.

Table 2–4 contains a breakdown of the number of incidents reported in terms of a numer of critical communication settings.

TABLE 2–4
Number of Critical Incidents Reported in
Four Life Areas

| LIFE AREA | NO. | % |
|---|---|---|
| Social | 493 | 43 |
| Family | 266 | 23 |
| Vocational | 256 | 23 |
| Social-Business | 124 | 11 |
| Total | 1139 | 100 |

E. M. Nett, L. G. Doefler, and J. Matthews, "The Relationship between Audiological Measures and Handicap," unpublished manuscript, Vocational Rehabilitation Administration, Project No. 167, 1960. Reprinted by permission.

For those who have worked with hard-of-hearing adults who are gradually losing their hearing, it is not surprising that the greatest number of incidents reported are in the area of social situations. It is here that they feel the greatest impact on their life-style. The social, family, and vocational categories are self-explanatory, but some discussion seems necessary regarding the social-business category. An example of this category is the situation one may find oneself in with a real estate agent. The agent is in the hearing-impaired person's home in a quasi-social atmosphere, but the purpose of the interaction has a purely business function.

Table 2–5 provides a breakdown of the number of incidents reported in each life area by the various respondents.

This table provides an excellent opportunity to see how hearing-impaired persons rank the categories in comparison with how those with whom they communicate daily rank them. It is important to note once again that hearing-impaired persons rank social situations high and that the greatest num-

TABLE 2–5
Number of Critical Incidents per Person Reporting
in Each Life Area, by Type of Respondent

| TYPE OF RESPONDENT | LIFE AREA | | | |
|---|---|---|---|---|
| | Social | Family | Vocational | Business-Social |
| Patient | 1.2 | .5 | 1.0 | .3 |
| Spouse | .5 | .7 | .0 | .1 |
| Relative | .5 | .4 | .0 | .1 |
| Friend | .8 | .0 | .0 | .1 |
| Coworker, Employer | .3 | .0 | 1.2 | .1 |

(Nett et al., p. 56. Reprinted by permission).

ber of incidents reported by all hearing-impaired respondents occurred in this category. Furthermore, both the hearing-impaired individuals and their employers agree on the importance of the vocational category.

Table 2–6 reports the type of problems reported in the life areas. The incidents were broken down primarily into four major categories: (1) those in which no auditory failure actually occurred; (2) those in which there was a failure to hear an auditory stimulus; (3) those in which there was a failure to understand or interpret speech or music; and (4) those in which there was a failure to localize an auditory stimulus. These categories were then broken down into more specific problems. The table shows the frequency with which these difficulties occurred in this group.

Approximately 70% of the incidents involved failure to understand speech or music, while only 20% involved failure to hear a stimulus. The fact that so many of the incidents reported centered around the problem of

TABLE 2–6
Type of Problems Reported in Critical Incidents

| TYPE OF PROBLEM | NO. | | % |
|---|---|---|---|
| Other than auditory failure | 80 | | 7 |
| Series of failures implied | | 78 | |
| Auditory illusion | | 2 | |
| Failure to hear stimulus | 239 | | 21 |
| Signal (bell, buzzer, bark) | | 80 | |
| Natural speech | | 151 | |
| Amplified speech or music | | 8 | |
| Failure to understand speech or music | 797 | | 70 |
| Natural speech | | 709 | |
| Amplified speech | | 88 | |
| Failure to localize sound | 23 | | 2 |
| Total | 1139 | | 100 |

(Nett et al., p. 57. Reprinted by permission).

TABLE 2-7
Type of Conditions of Failure

| CONDITIONS OF FAILURE | HEARING | | UNDER-STANDING | | LOCALI-ZATION | | TOTAL | |
|---|---|---|---|---|---|---|---|---|
| | No. | % | No. | % | No. | % | No. | % |
| Normal | 94 | 41 | 375 | 48 | 6 | 26 | 475 | 46 |
| Sound distractions | 20 | 9 | 95 | 12 | 1 | 4 | 116 | 11 |
| Auditorium | 11 | 5 | 94 | 12 | 1 | 4 | 106 | 10 |
| Intervening object | 49 | 21 | 38 | 5 | 2 | 9 | 89 | 9 |
| Unfavorable position | 26 | 11 | 50 | 7 | 2 | 9 | 78 | 8 |
| Insufficient volume | 7 | 3 | 67 | 9 | 0 | 0 | 74 | 7 |
| Acoustics | 16 | 7 | 26 | 3 | 11 | 48 | 53 | 5 |
| Distance across room | 6 | 2.5 | 23 | 3 | 0 | 0 | 29 | 3 |
| Tinnitus | 1 | 0.5 | 3 | 0.5 | 0 | 0 | 4 | 0.5 |
| Unfamiliar sounds | 0 | 0 | 4 | 0.5 | 0 | 0 | 4 | 0.5 |
| Total | 230 | 100 | 775 | 100 | 23 | 100 | 1028 | 100 |

(Nett et al., p. 58. Reprinted by permission).

understanding speech merely reinforces the need for audiologists to concentrate their aural rehabilitation efforts in this area.

Table 2–7 lists the type of conditions reported as auditory failures.

The largest number of failures occurred under normal sound conditions. The next largest categories were sound distractions and a distance as great as in an auditorium situation. This was especially true for problems of understanding. It is also interesting to note the substantial number of incidents reported that resulted from being in an unfavorable position or being obstructed by an intervening object. Difficulty in localizing was most often blamed on the acoustics of the room.

There is a significant relationship between the kind of auditory problem which a person reports and the social setting of the incident. Table 2–8 lists the social settings in which different types of auditory failures occur.

TABLE 2-8
Social Setting in which Different Types of Auditory Failures Occur

| SOCIAL SETTING | TYPES OF FAILURE | | | | | | | |
|---|---|---|---|---|---|---|---|---|
| | HEARING | | UNDER-STANDING | | LOCALI-ZATION | | TOTAL | |
| | No. | % | No. | % | No. | % | No. | % |
| Alone | 58 | 25 | 17 | 2 | 8 | 36 | 83 | 9 |
| Two-person group | 94 | 41 | 373 | 47 | 6 | 23 | 373 | 36 |
| Small informal group | 63 | 28 | 299 | 38 | 7 | 31 | 369 | 39 |
| Small formal group | 6 | 3 | 55 | 1 | 1 | 4 | 62 | 7 |
| Large formal group | 4 | 2 | 45 | 6 | 0 | 0 | 49 | 5 |
| Total | 225 | 99 | 789 | 100 | 22 | 94 | 936 | 96 |

(Nett et al., p. 58. Reprinted by permission).

Table 2–8 clearly shows that both hearing failures and understanding failures occur most often when the person is in a small informal group of two or more persons. Hearing failures also occur frequently when the person is alone, while understanding failures also occur fairly frequently in small or large formal groups. It is interesting to note that more auditory failures were reported as occurring in informal situations than in formal situations.

***Response to Auditory Failure.*** An interesting part of the University of Pittsburgh study consisted of asking the hearing-impaired subjects to report what they did when they experienced an auditory failure. Eleven separate responses, plus one combination of responses, were reported. These are listed in order of frequency of occurrence in Table 2–9.

TABLE 2–9
Response to Auditory Failure

| RESPONSE | NO. | % |
|---|---|---|
| Ask for repetition | 203 | 28 |
| Obtain assistance | 102 | 14 |
| Pretend, guess, or bluff | 98 | 14 |
| Intentionally do nothing | 89 | 12 |
| Get into a better position | 67 | 9 |
| Make a mechanical adaptation | 56 | 8 |
| Ask for repetition and get into | | |
| a better position | 28 | 4 |
| Withdraw | 27 | 4 |
| Tell about loss beforehand | 23 | 3 |
| Depend on sight | 17 | 2 |
| Read lips | 11 | 2 |
| Total | 721 | 100 |

(Nett et al., p. 60. Reprinted by permission).

With regard to the appropriateness of the responses made to the auditory failure condition, it would seem that the two responses reported most often (*ask for repetition* and *obtain assistance*) are excellent rehabilitative actions and suggestive of good adjustment to the situation. However, the next two most-often-reported responses (*pretend, guess, or bluff*, and *intentionally do nothing*) are certain to cause the hearing-impaired person problems. What is even more disturbing is how few people report using such perfectly good responses as *get into a better position, make a mechanical adaptation, ask for repetition and get into a better position, tell about loss beforehand,* and *depend on sight.*

Hearing-impaired subjects in the University of Pittsburgh study reported 290 incidents in which they were unable to respond at all to an auditory failure. What is most disturbing of all is that in 244 of these incidents the person was not even aware of the auditory failure until later and consequently was not in a position to correct the situation at the time it occurred.

As a result the subjects reported that they later learned that they had given incorrect responses to questions, had interrupted conversations, or had talked about subjects different from those under discussion. The remaining 46 incidents in which the hearing-impaired person did not respond occurred because someone else interceded (that is, answered the question addressed to the person, told someone he or she did not hear and asked for repetition, etc.).

○ HISTORY OF THE HEARING IMPAIRMENT

A number of psychological problems, communication problems, and unfavorable environmental conditions that may be experienced by persons with acquired hearing impairment have been discussed. The degree to which one or more of these conditions exists for a given hearing-impaired individual depends on a number of factors. Furthermore, the resulting hearing handicap is actually a function of a number of conditions that are often beyond the control of the hearing-impaired person. According to the report of the American Speech-Language-Hearing Association Task Force on the Definition of Hearing Handicap (1980),

> The degree to which a hearing impairment is a handicapping condition will depend on the interaction of a number of factors, and ideally any definition of hearing handicap should be based on a comprehensive consideration of the interrelationship of such factors as: the present age of the individual, the age of the individual when the impairment developed, the age of the person when the impairment was first discovered, the nature and extent of the hearing impairment, the person's communication needs and the nature of the settings in which communication occurs, the relationship of the hearing impairment to other physical or mental impairments, the amount and success of rehabilitative treatment already received, the individual's reaction and the reaction of others to his or her impaired hearing, and the effect of the hearing impairment on the individual's expressive communicative ability.*

It should become apparent that the identification and quantification of the handicapping effect of a given hearing impairment is a complex matter. Organic, psychological, and environmental parameters all play a role, with the weighting of each factor as yet unknown and most likely differing from person to person.

Sometimes tables and numbers do not convey the plight of a person experiencing an auditory failure. The manuscript of the University of Pittsburgh study included a number of verbatim accounts of incidents of audi-

*For the complete text of the report, see Appendix B.

tory failure from which many of the categories of response to auditory failure were drawn. These accounts are reproduced here to bring home the frustration and humiliation often experienced when one does not hear or understand what was said. The examples are drawn from the many incidents reported by the subjects to show how they were attempting to deal with their auditory failures (Nett et al 1960).

### asking for repetition.

Well, I was working what we call registered mail. . . . There are fellows on my left and right. We all stand up at the letter cages and work letters in the mail box. So I'd ask them a question, like if there is a certain post office in Pennsylvania that the mail has to go to. I'll ask them where is so-and-so. . . . They'll tell me but I actually won't hear them. I have to ask them two or three times. . . . When I don't understand what someone says to me I ask them what they said. Sometimes I have to ask two or three times. I feel guilty.

### obtaining assistance.

Well I went to H. E. Real Estate . . . when I got out of the service. We went to see about an apartment and I took my wife along because actually I knew I wouldn't be able to hear him anyway. . . . He started talking to me; I didn't hear a thing he was saying and I said, "Just a minute." I said to my wife, "Talk with him . . . and then you can sort of tell me.

It [the hearing loss] has dimmed the pleasure of the theatre particularly. It may be the acoustics. . . . The last time I went to the Nixon, I didn't get from under the balcony and on down and I was finished. I missed half the dialogue. I had to keep asking my wife what they said. So I won't go to a play unless I get the right seats.

### pretending.

I was at my brother's house last night. There was some conversation I didn't hear. I had to guess when to laugh. A couple of times I guessed wrong.

### doing nothing.

I have difficulty in Sunday school class. We have one class in each corner of the building and elsewhere. They're all having lessons at the same time. I sat in the second pew back of the teacher, facing him. A good many things I missed. . . . I just tried to catch as much as I could. And what I didn't get, I had to forget. I didn't want to interrupt others or disrupt the class.

### giving up.

Today at work all the fellows were eating lunch together. I just can't hear well in a bunch like that. I went over by myself and ate. . . . This happens almost every day.

**depending on sight.**
I just got my daughter a new bike. I have to keep checking on her all the time because I can't hear where she's at. This makes for extra steps. This happens all the time. She's only about 40 feet away when she's playing outside. . . . We're on a well-traveled road; they're doing quite a lot of building.

The purpose of this chapter is to introduce the reader to the plight of a considerable portion of the population who find themselves with hearing impairments of sufficient magnitude to affect their everyday living situations. The discussion began with the typical psychological problems often encountered in adjusting to the reality of the organic condition, moved to a discussion of the communication problems that are often experienced and the contribution of environmental conditions to these problems, and concluded with actual accounts by hearing-impaired persons of how their hearing impairments have affected aspects of their lives. The discussion centered on adults who lose their hearing after they have acquired their verbal communication skills and have completed most of their academic and vocational schooling. Special emphasis was given to those conditions which provide insight into the planning of rehabilitative programs.

It is hoped that the reader is convinced that this group of hearing-handicapped persons are in need of rehabilitative services and that these services must be improved. Indeed that is what is happening. Audiologist all over the world are reevaluating current audiological procedures with an eye toward making them more relevant to aural rehabilitation. The remainder of the book will be devoted to this endeavor.

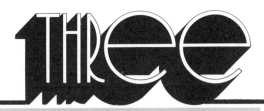

# Assessment of hearing handicap: audio-metric procedures

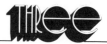

Clinical audiology plays a variety of roles in the rehabilitation of the hearing impaired. One of its key roles is to assess the effect of hearing impairment on the acquisition of language, as well as on educational, social, and verbal communication skills. If a hearing impairment is detected, three major concerns about the nature of the impairment typically emerge. The first concern deals with the reduction of energy or intensity of the perceived auditory message. This is referred to as the *extent of the hearing loss. Hearing loss* is defined as a loss of intensity, which is measured in decibels. The second concern deals with what *type of hearing disorder* is present. That is, whether it is primarily conductive, sensorineural, or the result of damage to some other site along the auditory pathway. Finally, the third concern is to investigate the degree to which the extent and type of the impairment combines with basic abilities and personality to cause a *handicapping effect.* Answers to these concerns contribute basic information for the planning of a significant portion of the rehabilitative process.

Information regarding these concerns can be obtained through the administration of one or a combination of several audiometric test procedures. These procedures can be categorized into three groups: (1) threshold measures; (2) suprathreshold measures; and (3) special tests, which combine a number of psychoacoustic measures. Each of these procedures will be discussed in terms of how it relates to the assessment of hearing handicap. A comprehensive discussion of these procedures and their role in the total clinical measurement of hearing impairment is beyond the scope of this chapter, and the reader is referred to Martin (1981) for review. However, from time to time modification of some procedures will be suggested to increase their clinical utility as tools for assessing hearing handicap.

The handicapping effect of auditory deprivation in adults has received considerably less attention from clinical audiologists than the areas of assessing extent and type of hearing impairment. One goal of this chapter is to alter this emphasis. Considerable information regarding handicap can be obtained from currently existing audiometric procedures by approaching these procedures from a slightly different perspective. This perspective places major emphasis on ascertaining the degree to which the hearing impairment has interfered with the communication process.

## ○ THRESHOLD MEASURES

As indicated earlier, one of the basic questions concerning the consequences of a given hearing impairment is how much intensity is lost from the perceived auditory message (i.e., What is the extent of the hearing loss?). It is generally believed that the extent of the hearing loss plays the most important role in determining how handicapping a hearing impairment is in crucial aspects of everyday living. This belief is supported by the numerous classification systems estimating handicap, educational placement, ability to understand speech, appropriate amplification (Davis and Silverman 1978), and social patterns (Vernon 1969). The standard audiological evaluation includes two basic threshold measures which assess the extent of the hearing loss: The first uses pure tones and the second uses speech signals. Each of these procedures will be discussed in terms of its contribution to assessing hearing handicap.

First, however, we must explore briefly the concept of *audiometric zero* in terms of medical diagnosis versus degree of handicap. With regard to medical diagnosis, a deviation of as little as 10 dB might be considered significant. On the other hand, degree of handicap must be defined in terms of sufficient deviation from audiometric zero to interfere with daily communication.

While audiometric zero is well established through laboratory methods and universally used, there is no generally accepted audiometric norm or reference level to define when a hearing loss becomes handicapping. However, audiometric zero may be viewed as an established starting point from which trained professionals begin to assess hearing in terms of hearing impairment (organic dysfunction) and hearing handicap (communication dysfunction). This differentiation will become much more evident when we discuss a number of threshold procedures used to classify hearing handicap.

### pure tone thresholds

Pure tone audiometry consists of presenting a series of calibrated pure tones at different frequencies and intensities to the listener by means of air and bone conduction. The goal is to determine the least (softest) amount of intensity needed to obtain a predetermined response to criteria. This is referred to as obtaining a listener's *pure tone threshold.* The measured threshold obtained for a given individual is typically compared to a standard established for persons with normal hearing as defined by the American National Standards Institute (ANSI) in 1969 and referred to as *audiometric zero.* The extent to which the listeners' thresholds vary from the standard for normal hearing is viewed as their hearing loss for that frequency. The average of the three critical frequencies (500, 1000, and 2000 Hz) is typically used to express the overall extent of the hearing loss.

Judgments regarding the handicapping effect of a particular impairment are often made on the basis of pure tone thresholds plotted on the audiogram as indicators of how much difficulty an individual might have in understanding everyday conversational speech. These judgments are most often made by (1) analyzing the *audiometric configuration* across all frequencies, (2) averaging the hearing thresholds of critical frequencies, and (3) computing the *percentage of hearing handicap* by one of several methods. While pure tone thresholds have their limitations in describing hearing handicap and must never be used alone to make this judgment, they do offer the trained audiologist considerable information and insight.

**Audiometric Configuration.** The audiometirc configuration represents an individual's hearing function in terms of the acoustic parameters of intensity (in relation to audiometic zero) and frequency. In terms of assessing hearing handicap, two questions can be asked on the basis of this information: (1) To what degree has conversational speech been rendered generally less audible?; (2) To what degree is it less intelligible? In other words, the audiometric configuration is often used to *predict* the degree to which a given individual will have difficulty *hearing* and *understanding* speech. Given that pure tones, rather than speech, have been used as the stimuli, the answers to these questions are actually predictions of handicap. However, in the hands of an audiologist with a solid background in the acoustics of speech production, speech perception, auditory coding and recoding, and hearing impairment, these observations can provide valuable information regarding the communication problems of a person.

For example, the extent to which the affected frequencies comprising the hearing impairment involve critical frequencies necessary to receive the spoken message will have a direct effect on (1) how much difficulty a given individual will have in being aware that someone is speaking to him or her, (2) how much difficulty he or she will have in understanding what is being said, or (3) a combination of both conditions. This is illustrated in Figures 3–1 and 3–2. Figure 3–1 represents a person with normal hearing in the lower audiometric test frequencies and reduced hearing in the higher frequencies beyond 2000 Hz. It is predicted that in a quiet setting this person will have little difficulty hearing and understanding what is being said. On the other hand, it is predicted that the person whose hearing is represented by the audiogram plotted in Figure 3–2 indicating that all audiometric frequencies are affected will experience difficulty in both hearing and understanding speech. As discussed in Chapter Two, the vowels, with low-frequency energy concentration, and the consonants, with high-frequency energy concentration, will both be affected, resulting in an intensity and speech intelligibility problem. This is only one example of how the audiometric configuration points to a number of potential communication prob-

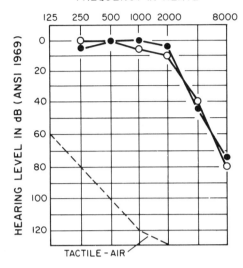

FREQUENCY IN HERTZ

FIGURE 3–1 Audiogram Illustrating Normal Hearing through 2000 Hz

lems which need further exploring. Other examples involve its use in hearing aid selection and potential speech deterioration.

*Classification of Hearing Handicap.* As a result of the obvious relationship between sensitivity for critical frequencies and hearing handicap (Davis and Silverman 1978; High et al. 1963) a number of handicap classification systems based on hearing threshold levels have been developed. Most of these systems are directed toward children and attempt to relate threshold levels to the successful acquisition of language, speech, educational, and verbal skills (Davis and Silverman 1978; Goetzinger 1978). These classification systems typially involve the averaging of 500, 1000, 2000, and sometimes 3000 and 4000 Hz to arrive at the upper and lower boundaries of each group within the classification.

The American Academy of Opthalmology and Otolaryngology (AAOO) proposed a classification system specifically designed for adults (Davis, 1965) to illustrate the relationship between hearing level, ability to understand speech, and degree of handicap. Six categories of hearing handicap were defined and are presented in Table 3–1. Each class is defined in terms of the average hearing level of three audiometric frequencies viewed as important for understanding speech. The classification system is based on the assumption that there is a close relationship between ability to understand conversational speech and the handicapping effect of a given hearing impairment. It is also assumed that it is possible to estimate a person's threshold for speech reasonably well from pure tone thresholds and that these threshold observations can predict general overall speech intel-

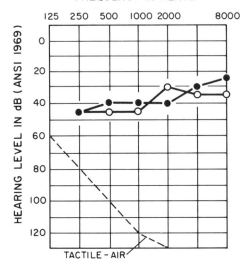

FREQUENCY IN HERTZ

FIGURE 3–2 Audiogram Illustrating
Reduced Hearing for All Frequencies

ligibility. The validity of this assumption will be addressed in a later section.

The classification system has many pitfalls. First, it is important to note that it was developed to compute workman's compensation and Veteran's Administration disability ratings (Davis and Silverman 1978). It applied primarily to persons having conductive hearing impairments with relatively flat audiometric configurations and persons having noise-induced hearing impairments. It does not take into account persons with poor speech discrimination or those who have the benefits of a hearing aid. Furthermore, the system does not consider the number of individual differences which hearing-impaired persons bring to the overall condition. Davis and Silverman write:

> With a given audiometric hearing threshold level, some persons will understand speech more easily and accurately, and others less easily and accurately, than is indicated in the table. Intelligence, quickness of perception, special training, general education, language background, motivation, ability to understand, and time of onset all contribute to the degree of an actual handicap. Any impairment of the central nervous system may greatly complicate the situation. Any one of several of these various factors may be vital in determining a person's overall economic or educational potentialities. (p. 269)

Most importantly, a number of arbitrary decisions were made regarding critical parameters of the classification system which seriously weaken its validity. Some of these arbitrary decisions include: (1) locating the point at which a hearing handicap begins (26 db HTL), (2) deciding what threshold

TABLE 3–1
Classes of Hearing Handicap
ISO = 1964

| dB | Class | Degree of Handicap | AVERAGE HEARING THRESHOLD LEVEL FOR 500, 1000, AND 1000 Hz IN THE BETTER EAR* | | Ability to Understand Speech |
|---|---|---|---|---|---|
| | | | More Than | Not More Than | |
| | A | Not significant | — | 25 dB (ISO) | No significant difficulty with faint speech |
| 25 | | | | | |
| | B | Slight handicap | 25 dB (ISO) | 40 dB | Difficulty only with faint speech |
| 40 | | | | | |
| | C | Mild handicap | 40 dB | 55 dB | Frequent difficulty with normal speech |
| 55 | | | | | |
| | D | Marked handicap | 55 dB | 70 dB | Frequent difficulty with loud speech |
| 70 | | | | | |
| | E | Severe handicap | 70 dB | 90 dB | Can understand only shouted or amplified speech |
| 90 | | | | | |
| | F | Extreme handicap | 90 dB | | Usually cannot understand even amplified speech |

*Whenever the average for the poorer ear is 25 dB or more greater than that of the better ear in this frequency range, 5 dB are added to the average for the better ear. This adjusted average determines the degree and class of handicap. For example, if a person's average hearing-threshold level for 500, 1000, and 2000 Hz is 37 dB in one ear and 62 dB or more in the other, his adjusted average hearing-threshold level is 42 dB and his handicap is Class C instead of Class B.

H. Davis, "Guide for the Classification and Evaluation of Hearing Handicap in Relation to Audiometric Zero," *Transactions of the American Academy of Opthamology and Otolaryngology*, Vol. 69 (1965), p. 741. Reprinted by permission.

levels comprise a maximum handicap (92 dB HTL), and (3) developing the descriptive statements labeling the degree of handicap and the ability to understand speech. These descriptive statements do not take into account the qualitatively different hearing demands of educational and employment settings. Also, the choice of frequencies used to compute the averages is now under considerable question. These objections will be discussed later.

In an attempt to improve on the AAOO system, the armed services developed a system of hearing threshold profiles that were based on predetermined sensitivity requirements associated with various job tasks. These profiles are presented in Table 3-2 and represent a considerable improvement over the AAOO classifications in that they attempt to weigh hearing thresholds and the number of frequencies considered as a function of job tasks. They have also included frequencies above 2000 Hz in their computations, and these frequencies have been found to have an effect on speech intelligibility, especially in noisy conditions which are often found in many normal listening situations.

TABLE 3-2
Acceptable Audiometric Hearing Levels (ANSI Scale)

A. *For Appointment, Enlistment, and Induction*

| | | 500 | 1000 | 2000 | 4000 Hz |
|---|---|---|---|---|---|
| (a) | Both ears | average of these three frequencies not over 30 dB with no one of them over 35 dB | | | 55 |
| | or | | | | |
| (b) | Better ear | 30 | 25 | 25 | 35 |
| | Worse ear | | no requirement | | |

B. *Physical Profile Functional Capacity Guide*

| Profile serial | | 500 | 1000 | 2000 | 4000 Hz |
|---|---|---|---|---|---|
| 1 | Each ear | | average not over 25 dB | | not over 45 |
| 2 | Both ears | | average not over 30 dB | | not over 55 |
| | Better ear | | average not over 25 dB | | not over 35 |
| 3 | | may have hearing level at 30 dB with hearing aid by speech-reception | | | |
| 4 | | score below retention standard | | | |

C. *Medical Fitness Standard for Mobilization*

Hearing: Uncorrected hearing, average level at 500, 1000, and 2000 Hz, of 40 dB or more is unfitting for service

D. *Mediocodenial Registrants*

Hearing: Hearing which cannot be improved in one ear with a hearing aid to an average hearing level of 30 dB or less in the speech-reception range is a cause of medical unfitness; unilateral deafness is not disqualifying

Adapted from *Army Regulations* "AR 40-501 Medical Service Standards of Medical Fitness," (Dec. 1969), Appendix 2, Tables 1–3. Reprinted by permission of office of The Surgeon General, Department of the Army, DASG-PSP, Washington, DC 20310.

***Percentage of Hearing Handicap.*** A second part of the AAOO classification system includes a procedure for computing a *percentage of hearing handicap*; it was originally described by AAOO in 1965 and was revised in 1979. This procedure consists of averaging the hearing thresholds of four critical frequencies (500, 1000, 2000, and 3000 Hz), assigning a 1.5 percentage value for each dB of diminished hearing after 25 dB (ANSI 1969) with a maximum of 92 dB, and computing a percentage of hearing handicap for each ear separately. The binaural percentage of hearing handicap is computed by multiplying the percentage of the better ear by 5, adding the percentage of the poorer ear, and dividing by 6. The rationale and complete directions for computing the AAOO percentage of hearing handicap may be found in Appendix A.

A number of criticisms have been made of the AAOO approaches to classification of handicap and percentage of hearing handicap. One deals with the appropriate HL of 26 dB (re. ANSI 1969) for the low fence. There is sufficient evidence that the relationship between pure tone thresholds and speech intelligibility is frequency dependent (Kryter 1973; Suter 1977); and the lower boundary of 26 dB, using 500, 1000, 2000, and 3000 Hz as suggested by AAOO, may be inappropriate. Similar concern over the other end of the continuum is also expressed. A high fence of 92 dB (re. ANSI 1969) is considered much too severe. Even loud conversational speech would not be sustained at levels much over 80 dB for any length of time, and it is unreasonable to assume that the handicap is not severe until hearing thresholds exceed 92 dB. While the inclusion of 3000 Hz, as suggested in the 1979 revision, improves the potential for identifying persons who will experience difficulty in noisy listening conditions (Kryter 1963; Harris 1965; Suter 1977), retaining 500 Hz as part of the average may well be counterproductive.

Most importantly, the major criticism of the system concerns the rationale for converting pure tone thresholds into percentage points which express handicap. The rationale has never been adequately argued in the literature and remains in fact artificial and arbitrary. Similarly, the choice of any numerical value to describe growth of handicap as a function of averaged hearing thresholds is also clearly arbitrary. The rationale for the weighting procedure for computing percentage of hearing handicap for bilateral hearing impairments is also unclear and is considered inappropriate by some (Macrae 1976).

Finally, there is considerable discrepancy between the percentage of hearing handicap values and other assessments of hearing handicap. In addition to the problems cited in the literature (Macrae 1976; Kell et al. 1971; Noble 1970; Atherly and Noble 1971), most clinicians have repeatedly experienced the inadequacies of pure tone thresholds for describing actual listening behavior. The situation of two hearing-impaired persons with nearly identical audiograms and grossly diverse behavioral symptoms is commonly observed in clinical settings.

The American Speech, Language, and Hearing Association Task Force on the Definition of Hearing Handicap prepared a report in 1980 which represents a fairly concise review of the history of such procedures and a critical analysis of their computational process. It offers a revised approach which is more reasonable than any other percentage of hearing handicap procedure currently being used. Because of the importance of recognizing the limitations of such procedures, the report is reproduced in Appendix B.

### speech reception threshold (SRT)

As suggested in the previous section, the degree to which a hearing impairment interferes with the ability to receive and understand conversational speech can be used as an indication of hearing handicap. While the audiometric configuration and the average of selected pure tone thresholds offer considerable insight into speech reception and intelligibility, they are only predictive. A more direct measure of these skills can be obtained by using speech rather than pure tones as the auditory signal. *Speech audiometry* was developed to obtain this measure.

The clinical value of speech audiometry, which allows for systematic presentation of carefully selected speech stimuli through a calibrated communication system, is not always fully realized. This chapter will expand the use of the *speech reception threshold* (SRT) and the *speech discrimination score* (SDS) beyond their historical roles.

The speech reception threshold measure will be discussed as part of this section, and the suprathreshold measure of speech discrimination will be covered in the following section. In accordance with the purpose of this chapter, both procedures will only be discussed in terms of how they offer information useful in assessing hearing handicap.

The SRT is typically obtained by presenting a series of words, either live voice or recorded, through an electrical system that controls intensity. The intensity at which the words are presented is progressively reduced until threshold is reached. The most common clinical test items are standardized lists of disyllabic words (spondees) that can be spoken with equal stress as monitored through the use of a volume unit meter.

***Clinical Application.*** It should be stated at the outset that the role of the SRT in assessing hearing handicap is primarily to provide corroborative and base-line information for additional testing. In addition, however, in cases of difficult-to-test persons such as some elderly patients or those with suddenly acquired hearing impairments, the SRT can offer worthwhile information in conjunction with other audiologic data.

One of the basic questions concerning the consequences of a given hearing impairment is how much intensity is lost from the perceived auditory message (i.e., What is the extent of the hearing loss?). The SRT estimates the extent of the hearing loss for speech. Threshold is the point at which a listener can repeat 50% of the speech message presented to him. Threshold measures for speech are highly reliable (Tillman and Jerger 1959) and can easily be obtained from a variety of listeners as long as they can follow instructions or be taught to recognize a picture of the test item and to indicate that recognition.

Consequently, one of the obvious values of the SRT is its close relation to pure tone thresholds, especially those used to comprise the standard pure tone average. This corroborative role is an important one, especially in cases where inconsistent pure tone responses were obtained. Because the listener must hear enough of the test word to repeat it correctly, the likelihood of false positive response is greatly reduced.

Furthermore, in cases of some elderly or mentally ill persons or persons with severe hearing losses, where pure tone thresholds and suprathresholds for speech are difficult to obtain, the SRT or some modification of the procedure may well enhance the information available regarding the extent of hearing loss and how speech is being processed. Some of these modifications include obtaining a *speech awareness threshold,* restricting the word list, pretraining with the word list to enhance familiarization, and using oversimplified instructions given in briefer time units and repeated more often.

Because response to the SRT procedure and some of its modified forms is sometimes more successful than response to suprathreshold speech measures, the degree to which the SRT approximates the pure tone air conduction audiometric configuration can offer some insight into how well the reduced hearing is used. Returning to Figure 3-1, the person with this audiogram and an SRT of **5dB HL** could be viewed as using available communication cues more efficiently than a second person with the same audiogram and a much worse SRT. While this kind of information is more easily deduced from suprathreshold speech measures, the SRT procedure is mentioned here as an alternative approach when the preferred measures are not obtainable.

The most important contribution of the SRT to assessing hearing handicap is that it provides a base line from which to assess the listener's performance with speech materials presented under various conditions at suprathreshold levels. The importance of this base line will emerge more fully in the following section on suprathreshold measures.

○ SUPRATHRESHOLD MEASURES

Information about the listener's response to auditory stimuli at suprathreshold levels is also quite useful. Because of the close relationship between speech intelligibility and hearing handicap, the bulk of the discussion will deal with those measures employing speech at suprathreshold levels. However, the role of suprathreshold procedures employing pure tones will also be considered.

### speech discrimination testing

For normal hearing listeners, conversational speech does not occur at threshold levels, but rather at suprathreshold levels. Difficulty in perceiving speech at these suprathreshold levels will most certainly influence general communication efficiency. Speech discrimination testing was originally designed to measure the listener's ability to repeat a speech message which is presented at an intensity known to yield a high performance score from listeners with normal hearing. One of the most common procedures employed in a typical audiologic diagnostic setting is to obtain a *maximum intelligibility score* using one of several monosyllabic word lists presented at 30 dB to 40 dB SL. This measure has been referred to historically as a *speech discrimination score* and is defined as the point at which increased intensity does not produce an improved intelligibility score.

The speech intelligibility measure using the traditional maximum intelligibility concept, which encompasses a single message and presentation level, has turned out to be quite limiting in terms of its original goal. Its major clinical value lies in its role in differentiating between cochlear, re-trocochlear, and central auditory lesions. However, the basic concept of speech audiometry, the use of ability to understand everyday conversational speech as in indication of hearing handicap, is still viable. An expanded view of this concept allows the audiologist to use speech in various forms and to present it at several intensity levels and under a number of different listening conditions. With this expanded view, the potential of speech audiometry as an assessment of communication problems associated with hearing impairment is quite good, and it can be used to assess a number of parameters of hearing handicap.

*Conversational Speech.* Speech audiometry provides an opportunity for direct assessment of difficulty experienced in understanding everyday conversational speech under various listening conditions. A preselected speech message can be presented through earphones to each ear separately in quiet conditions or in a sound field. The message may be presented in quiet conditions at normal conversational intensity levels, as well as at levels which represent soft speech or loud speech. Further investigation could include presenting equivalent speech materials at the same stimulus input levels in a sound field with competing noise (Carhart, 1969; Olsen and Carhart 1967; Olsen and Tillman 1968; Tillman et al. 1970). This noisy environment test situation should provide an assessment of the listener's performance when the primary signal is directly in front of the listener and the competing message is on either or both sides, or when the primary signal is on one side and the competing message is on the other side. These decisions will depend upon the hearing loss in each ear and the ear being considered for a hearing aid. In either case the question, How well does the listener follow everyday conversational speech? is being assessed in both a quiet and a noisy environment.

In addition to assessing the listener's performance with auditory cues alone, one should assess the listener's performance with visual cues added. The degree to which visual cues are used contributes much to identifying specific problems and assists in selecting rehabilitative activities (Erber 1971a; Erber 1971b; Erber 1972). For example, knowing that a listener yields an extremely poor score when a speech message is presented with no visual cues but a considerably higher score when visual cues are added offers information about how much the listener is using his or her residual hearing. Depending on the extent of the hearing loss, this will guide the clinician in planning the appropriate auditory training program. A visual message by itself will also offer additonal information (Hutton, Curry, and Armstrong 1959). Ross et al. (1972) found that the combined visual auditory (look-listen) measure produced a higher score than adding the auditory alone (listen) score to the visual alone (look) score or subtracting the auditory alone (listen) score from the score for a combined discrimination message in a standard lip-reading test. There should be two equal forms so that pretest and posttest measures can be taken following a systematic treatment program. This would also provide information on performance with connected speech.

*Hearing Aids.* Appropriate amplification plays an important role in minimizing the handicapping effects of hearing impairment. While there are several points of view presented in the literature concerning various procedures for hearing aid evaluation and selection (Carhart 1950; Shore et al. 1960; Resnick and Becker 1963), almost all agree that speech audiometry plays an important role in facilitating appropriate amplification. One reason is that unaided and aided responses to speech can be obtained in a sound field listening setting, and this enables the clinician to evaluate the listener's performance with and without an aid and to compare performance among aids. A discussion of the various amplification selection procedures described in the literature is beyond the scope of this chapter. However, this writer believes that aided measurements for the purpose of choosing appropriate amplification should include (1) measurements with speech at conversational and tolerance levels and (2) measurements with competing messages. With varying degrees of success, a competent audiologist employing speech audiometry can rule out inappropriate amplification units and delineate hearing aids with amplification adequate to the user. These procedures are far superior to selecting hearing aids exclusively on the basis of audiograms and factory specifications describing the hearing aids' physical amplification characteristics.

*Auditory Training.* An indication of how well the listener will respond to auditory training can be obtained through speech audiometry. By using a closed-set response mode and an aided conversational-level stimulus input, the clinician can determine how well the listener should learn to use his or her residual hearing after a brief training period in the test booth. For example, the listener can be presented with a number of words in written or picture form and given a number of trials to identify these words when both visual and auditory cues are offered. The visual cues can then be removed to see if any generalization to auditory alone has taken place. The set of choices in both the brief training period and the test situation can consist of a two-, four-, or six-choice response set. This procedure is by no means an auditory training program, but it is a procedure the audiologist can perform in a diagnostic setting, and it may offer rehabilitative information beyond the traditional SDS.

The procedure suggested above also argues for pretraining with test words prior to the testing session. There is no question that a threshold more dependent on intensity changes can be obtained with this approach. A similar pretraining approach is suggested in suprathreshold speech testing and is actually included in some test procedures with normally hearing children (Goldman, Fristoe, and Woodcock 1970). The rationale for such an approach is to minimize vocabulary deficiency as an influencing factor and to more closely test speech discrimination. An excellent discussion of the use of such an approach with severely hearing-impaired persons is found in Lloyd (1972).

*Clinical Value.* Speech audiometry has been discussed as a valuable tool for assessing hearing handicap by investigating a person's performance with speech messages. It was pointed out that its value is greatly enhanced when the clinical questions go beyond the traditional maximum intelligibility score. The following procedures will maximize the clinical value of speech audiometric tests: (1) carefully selecting the speech message (monosyllabic word lists, sentences, etc.); (2) varying the intensity presentation level (above, below, and at conversational levels); (3) including both quiet and noisy listening conditions; and (4) testing with and without visual cues. If these steps are taken, a considerable amount of information may be gained regarding a person's performance in everyday listening situations.

The number and nature of the clinical questions asked will vary from patient to patient and will depend greatly on the time available with the patient. Following are three questions that may be helpful in obtaining insight into the handicapping effect of a particular hearing impairment.

1. *Speech Message. Does a person's speech intelligibility score differ from what might be expected when various speech messages are used* (Epstein et al. 1968)? For example, if a person's score does not improve appreciably when sentences are used which offer considerably more contextual cues than would be offered by a list of unrelated isolated words, the person is considerably more handicapped than if the reverse were true. This suggests that there may be problems not only in the peripheral mechanisim, but in central auditory processing.

2. *Intensity Presentation Level. What kinds of difficulty does a person experience when speech is presented softly, at conversational level, or somewhat loudly?* Performance at these levels offers obvious information regarding the need and specific use of amplification. The person with poor speech intelligibility at conversational level is obviously quite handicapped and may be in need of hearing aid. A person may have excellent speech intelligibility scores at conversational and above conversational levels and poor scores at slightly below conversational levels, but if that person's typical listening conditions are such that people speak quietly, he or she may also be a candidate for amplification. On the other hand, a person with similar scores but different listening conditions may not need amplification at all.

3. *Visual Cues versus Auditory Cues. Does a person's speech intelligibility score vary considerably when visual cues are added to auditory cues with equiva-*

*lent speech messages?* The person who improves considerably when visual cues are added is clearly less handicapped than the person whose score does not improve appreciably. Very different rehabilitative procedures are in order for the latter person.

The typical reaction to suggestions such as those above is that there is simply not sufficient time in a standard audiological test session to conduct the additional testing. This is true. The place for this kind of testing is not in the initial diagnostic setting but in subsequent sessions, and it is only appropriate for those persons for whom audiological rehabilitation involves amplification and communication skills programs.

### social adequacy index

One attempt to use both the SRT and the SDS to arrive at an estimate of social hearing effectiveness is the *social adequacy index* (SAI) (Davis 1948). The SAI estimates social adequacy in terms of ability to follow everyday conversational speech. It is based on the ability to identify words on speech intelligibility tests presented at three standard hearing levels for conversational speech: faint (33 dB), average (48 dB), and loud (63 dB). Thus, the SAI is the mean of the discrimination scores obtained at each of the three standard levels of intensity. A table from which the SAI can be computed has been devised, and the clinician need only determine the SRT and obtain the maximum intelligibility score binaurally to arrive at a person's SAI (Davis 1948).

The SAI has not received wide clinical use. Davis and Silverman (1978) commented on the reasons:

> Actually, the idea has not worked out very well. One reason is that the PB recordings never have been standardized well enough to measure a man's discrimination with anything like the accuracy that we measure his threshold level. Also, we do not yet seem to know quite enough about the relation of the hearing and understanding of connected speech in words and sentences to its component frequencies, phonemes, and syllables.

The SAI may overestimate difficulty in understanding ordinary conversational speech (Giolas 1966b). The Giolas study, however, used normally hearing subjects listening to a distorted message. Studies using hearing-handicapped persons demonstrated a relationship between the SAI and meaures of handicap which describe actual problem areas. High, Fairbanks, and Glorig (1964) found a close correlation between the SAI and a self-administered scale measuring handicap. It is interesting to note that no correlation was found between the self-administered scale and the SDS obtained with the W-22 word list. Similarly, Nett, Doerfler, and Mathews

(1960) found that the SAI was predictive of scores on all the tests which they developed. It appears that the SAI, utilizing both sensitivity and discrimination measures, may be a more valid estimate than its minimal use implies.

A few comments should be made regarding the appropriate speech message to be used in suprathreshold measures. The literature contains reliability data and, to a lesser degree, validity data regarding many speech messages typically used. However, these data, often offered as norms, are based on the data generated from specific recordings of the speech message being used as the test stimulus. With a few exceptions most of these recordings are not commercially available. On the other hand, a speech audiometric test is an acoustic event consisting of a given speaker, a recording procedure, a specific form of message degradation (if one is used), and a scoring procedure. It is inappropriate to use the written form of the speech stimuli, administer them in a recorded or live-voice version, and assume the same reliability and validity constraints imposed by the original recordings.

However, from the standpoint of assessing hearing handicap, the lack of these norms and standardized recordings and procedures takes on a lesser importance. By systematically varying the (1) message, (2) presentation level, (3) method of message degradation, and (4) use of visual cues, the knowledgeable and experienced clinician can piece together a fairly clear picture of a given person's speech perception pattern. Even without standard norms, much can be learned by comparing the same person's performance under different conditions.

With regard to specific speech messages, the following guidelines are offered. The material may be administered live voice or recorded, and the clients may be used as their own norm.

1. The CID W-22 monosyllabic word lists recorded by Hirsh tend to yield the highest scores regardless of hearing loss, and more of a hearing loss is required to secure a reduced (less than 90%) score.

2. The Harvard Psycho-Acoustic Laboratory (PAL) PB-50 monosyllabic word lists, as recorded by Rush Hughes, contain many unfamiliar words, and less of a hearing loss is necessary to obtain a lowered SDS. Normals have been found to yield a score no better than 88% (Giolas and Epstein 1963). These word lists are considerably more sensitive to the discrimination difficulty presented by persons with a sensorineural hearing impairment. Accordingly, Silverman and Hirsh (1955) have suggested that clinicians return to the use of the Rush Hughes recordings for this kind of diagnostic information. Lower scores will also be obtained with live-voice or rerecorded versions of these lists.

3. Scores on the Northwestern monosyllabic word lists seem to fall in between those on the CID and Harvard PB-50 word lists. This impression is based on clinical observations of scores obtained with our recordings; these observations are consistent with those reported by Tillman and Carhart (1966).

There are those who feel that a larger unit of speech, such as a sentence or even some form of quantifiable continuous discourse, is more appropriate (Berger 1969; Giolas 1966a; Harris, Haines, and Myers 1960; Kalico et al., 1977; Speaks and Jerger 1965). Sentences present a more natural listening task; they enable the subject to take advantage of crucial parameters used in understanding connected speech. Several sentence lists have been developed to measure speech discrimination; however, they have not received general clinical use. Theoretical arguments and empirical data strongly suggest that their use is long overdue. The CID sentence lists (Silverman and Hirsh 1955) have been suggested as one possible message for clinical and research use. They were developed to be representative of colloquial speech, and a close relationship has been found between scores obtained using selected CID sentence lists. The lists in this series are available in written form (Davis and Silverman 1978) and are easy to administer and score. Harris et al. (1960) have revised the lists in an attempt to provide a greater homogeneity of sentence length while maintaining the colloquial speech pattern. These lists are known as the revised CID sentence lists (R-CID). Neither of these sentence lists is available in commercially recorded form, and their list equivalency has not been established (Giolas and Duffy 1973). Other sentence lists include the multiple choice series developed by Berger (1969) and the synthethic sentences proposed by Speaks and Jerger (1965). In spite of some fairly impressive data supporting the clinical use of some of these sentence lists (Jerger 1973), they have not been incorporated into the routine battery of speech tests.

## ○ SPECIAL AUDIOMETRIC PROCEDURES

A number of additional auditory tests have been developed to measure a listener's ability to (1) make loudness judgments (loudness balance procedures); (2) sustain a continuous and interrupted pure tone (Bekesy audiometry, low-and-high level tone decay); (3) detect 1 dB amplitude changes of specific pure tones (short increment sensitivity index); and (4) respond to impedance and acoustic reflex measures. Along with pure tone and speech audiometry and a thorough otological evaluation and case history, these tests assist in identifying the type of hearing impairment. Each of these measures offers information as to the potential success of remedial procedures such as surgery, medicine, and amplification and determines the need for follow-up audiological and otological services. It has been suggested that diagnostic categories such as conductive and sensorineural hearing impairment play a major role in planning specific aural rehabilitation programs. These categories are certainly important for medical diagnosis and treatment. However, from the standpoint of delineating specific problems experienced by the individual with the hearing difficulty for purposes of planning rehabilitative activities, these categories are prognostic rather than diagnostic. A person with 40 dB sensorineural hearing loss could have any combination of several communication problems usually associated with this diagnostic category, and further evaluation is necessary to determine the person's actual hearing handicap. Attempts to assign a diagnostic label may actually serve to obscure the deficit behaviors rather than pinpoint them (McReynolds 1967). The set of behavior patterns usually associated with a particular diagnostic category is often imposed on persons being evaluated rather than used as a checklist with which to evaluate how well they fit the expected model. In medically nonreversible hearing impairments, information obtained after a rehabilitation program has begun is often more valuable than previously assigned diagnostic categories. Observable behavioral symptoms often associated with clinical categories such as conductive or sensorineural hearing impairments must only be used as general guidelines for further investigation and not as independent diagnostic indices of communication problems.

Traditional audiologic test procedures have been discussed in this chapter in terms of their contribution to assessing hearing handicap. It has been pointed out repeatedly that these procedures provide considerable information with regard to how a particular hearing impairment manifests itself as a communication problem. Clinical audiologists have been encouraged to expand their view of these procedures to include, with some test administration modifications, their role as guides to rehabilitative activities. It has also been stressed that these modifications are only appropriate when concerns emerge regarding handicap. It is this author's contention that these concerns usually emerge after the initial diagnostic setting, when it becomes apparent that the hearing impairment is nonmedically reversible and that further audiological decisions are in order. When this is the case, the hearing handicap and the resulting communication problems become concerns, and it becomes appropriate to pursue additional audiological procedures such as those that have been discussed in this chapter.

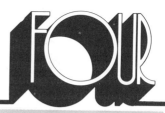

# Assessment of hearing handicap: self-report procedures

The *handicapping* effect of hearing impairment has been stressed throughout the first three chapters of this book. Chapter Three established the *assessment* of hearing handicap as an important function of the audiologist and described the degree to which audiometric procedures provide information along these lines. This chapter will introduce some of the limitations of audiometric procedures as measures of hearing handicap and develop a rationale for using the *self-report* approach in identifying the communication problems associated with a given person's hearing impairment.

It is generally accepted that audiologic test procedures which measure the ear's response to calibrated auditory stimuli in a controlled setting provide considerable information regarding the extent and type of hearing impairment. On the other hand, there is less satisfaction with the degree to which these procedures provide concrete information regarding how a given hearing impairment has influenced a specific person's life situation in general and verbal communication in particular (Noble 1978; Giolas 1970). Noble (1978) suggests that audiometric procedures are at worst misleading and at best inadequate when they are used as predictors of hearing handicap.

Most clinicians have had the experience of dealing with two hearing-impaired persons with quite *similar* audiograms and quite *dissimilar* communication problems or with a person who has a low speech discrimination score obtained in the traditional manner but who reports minimal communication difficulty.

One explanation for these discrepancies lies in the target behaviors measured by audiologic procedures (Noble 1978). These procedures measure the ear's response to specific auditory stimuli (pure tones, selected speech messages, etc.) in a laboratory setting (quiet and simulated noisy conditions). The clinician is required to infer from these results the person's performance in typical listening-speaking situations. The accuracy of these inferences depends upon how representative these laboratory conditions are of the everyday communication setting. As discussed in Chapter Two, the communication process is not only dependent upon the ear's physical status (organic impairment), but is also quite dependent upon a number of factors such as: (1) with whom the person is speaking (relationship to the speaker); (2) under what conditions the communication act is occurring (number of speakers, environmental noise conditions); and (3) the purpose of the verbal intercourse (social, work, business). Consequently, it has become apparent that audiometric procedures as they are typically administered are not representative of most listening-speaking situations and as a result generate only general and predictive statements regarding how a person will function in most real-world communication situations. For example, audiometric procedures can suggest difficulty with the loudness of the signal or probable difficulty with understanding speech even when it is made comfortably loud, but they fall quite short of describing when, where, and with whom these communication problems typically occur for the person being tested. Furthermore, they offer no information regarding how the person feels about having a hearing impairment. The clinician must have this information if the total rehabilitative process is to be optimally effective. The modified audiometric procedures described in Chapter Two go a long way toward correcting the almost exclusively prognostic nature of such procedures, but they still leave the clinician with more unknowns than knowns. What is needed is an approach to assessing hearing performance that yields data which is more than predictive. In 1970, Giolas wrote:

> Today, the most widely used source for obtaining information of this type is the rehabilitation program itself. Through observation and discussion, over a period of time, areas of difficulty are determined. When this is accomplished, a program to meet specific needs can be established. However, this process is time consuming, and until a person's particular problems are identified the treatment program can be only minimally effective. A standard procedure for obtaining this information early is needed. (p. 2)

Renewed interest in assessing hearing handicap by other than audiometric procedures has resulted in the development of several self-report procedures which show promise in achieving this goal.

## ○ THE SELF-REPORT APPROACH

Among the major responsibilities of clinical audiologists are: (1) assessing the handicapping effects of hearing impairment, especially in terms of communication, and (2) gauging the success of any rehabilitative process (medical or nonmedical) in terms of alleviating or minimizing these handicapping effects. The inadequacies of audiometric measures in identifying actual problem areas experienced in real-world listening-speaking situations were discussed in Chapter Three and the preceding section of this chapter. Associated with these inadequacies is the added problem of using these same procedures to initiate and assess gains made as a result of aural rehabilitation programs. To accomplish this, the procedures must address issues that lend themselves to specific management activities. The psychophysical audiometric measures, which are primarily designed to assess the organic status of the auditory mechanism, assess target behaviors which do not lend themselves to management activities. Even if speech and/or pure tone measures are improved as a result of amplification, the information provided by these measures is at best quite general and has variable predictability with regard to generalizing to specific communication situations for a given person.

The behaviors which are expected to improve after rehabilitative intervention and which should be the object of assessment tools are (1) the behaviors comprising the communication process (as described in Chapter Two) and (2) the coping strategies used by the hearing-impaired person.

In an attempt to more closely align the measuring tools with the appropriate behaviors to be assessed, a number of new self-report instruments for general clinical use have been developed over the past fifteen years. The basic format of these scales consists of presenting the hearing-impaired person with a series of questions centering around a potentially handicapping condition and asking the person to judge his or her overall performance in specific situations. The following sample question is taken from the hearing handicap scale developed by High, Fairbanks, and Glorig (1964).

> Can you hear adequately when you are conversing with more than one person?
> ———Practically always.
> ———Frequently.
> ———As often as not.
> ———Occasionally.
> ———Almost never.

The major differences between most of these instruments lie in purpose; scope; number of items comprising the questionnaire; and, in some cases, test administration and scoring. An in-depth discussion of each of these instruments is beyond the scope of this book; however, Tables 4-1 and 4-2 summarize some of the salient characteristics of those procedures developed since 1964 which have been offered for clinical use. The reader is encouraged to review these tests in the event that one or more fit the particular needs of his or her work setting and case load. The reader is also encouraged to read Part III of Dr. W. Noble's book, *Assessment of Impaired Hearing* (1978), for an in-depth critical analysis of most self-report procedures, including some earlier attempts at nonscaled inventories.

On the other hand, four of these instruments have particular significance in guiding the development of the self-report approach as it currently exists and warrant discussion in somewhat more detail.

### hearing handicap scale

The most familiar self-report instrument used for assessing hearing handicap is the *Hearing Handicap Scale* (HHS) developed by High, Fairbanks, and Glorig (1964). The HHS consists of two forms of twenty items each. The questions represent several common communication situations, including listening on the telephone and listening in the presence of background noise. The respondents are asked to rate the frequency with which they believe they experience difficulty in the situation described. A five-point scale is provided identical to the one in the sample question presented in the preceding section. The total point values for all responses are obtained and a single percentage score is calculated to signify degree of handicap.

A number of studies have been conducted comparing scores obtained on the HHS and on standard audiometric measures. The major findings conclude that the HHS scores are: (1) closely related to sensitivity measures such as the Pure Tone Average (Jerger et al. 1968; Speaks et al. 1970; Noble and Atherly 1970); (2) moderately related to selected speech discrimination scores obtained with an elderly population (Blumenfeld et al. 1969; Berkowitz and Hochberg 1971); and (3) somewhat related to type of hearing impairment (Blumenfeld et al. 1969; Noble and Atherly 1970).

The major limitation of the HHS lies in its narrow scope. It was designed to yield a single number that would suggest the overall magnitude of handicap. Furthermore, the final items selected to comprise the two forms leaned heavily on hearing sensitivity difficulties, which probably explains the close relationship between scores obtained on the HHS and audiometric threshold measures. At the same time, the HHS was the first instrument to attend to some long-needed test design rigors such as test-retest reliability, and it served as the major impetus for further research in this area. At the present time the HHS still represents the quickest standard procedure which a clinician can use to obtain some idea of the communication difficulties the hearing-impaired person identifies as problematic. In addition, the good split-half reliability between Forms A and B lends itself quite readily to research. A complete copy of the HHS can be found in Appendix C.

### hearing measurement scale

The *Hearing Measurement Scale* (HMS) developed by Noble and Atherly (1970) represents an important step in the renewed interest in assessing hearing handicap with self-report procedures. It introduced into the literature an instrument with a considerably expanded scope compared with that of the Hearing Handicap Scale. Noble and Atherly (1970), in noting that the subjects used to develop the Hearing Handicap Scale did not include a broad representation of hearing disorders, expressed a need for

TABLE 4–1
Description Data and Selected Statistical Results of Studies Examining
Instruments for Self-Assessment of Hearing Handicap

| Study | Handicap Scale | N | Mean Age | Age Range | Description of Subjects | Test Ear | Mean Scale Score | Scale Score Range |
|---|---|---|---|---|---|---|---|---|
| High et al. 1964 | HHS-A and B | 50 | 49 | 21–72 | Mostly conductive or mixed | Better Poorer | A-45% B-45% | NA |
| Blumenfeld et al. 1969 | HHS-A HHS-B | 46 | 59 | 27–82 | | Left | NA | NA |
| Speaks et al. 1970 | HHS-A | 60 | 59 | 19–78 | Mostly sensorineural | Better | 42% | 6-100% |
| Berkowitz and Hochberg 1971 | HHS-A | 100 | 70 | 60–87 60–89 70–79 80–89 | All sensorineural | Better | 45% 44% 45% 56% | NA |
| Peters 1974 | HHS-A HHS-B HHS-A and B comb. | 40 | 49 | 19–65 | Male VA patients, sensorineural | — | 65% 64% | (94) (89) |
| McCartney et al. 1976 | HHS-A | 36 | 75 | 62–89 | Mostly sensorineural | Better | 42% | 10-90% |
| Kuller 1976 | HHS-B | 40 | 83 | 67–108 | Sensorineural | Better | 61% | 23-100% |
| Schow and Tannahill 1977 | HHS-B | 50 | 46 | 18–88 | Normal and sensorineural | NA | 30% | 0-96% |
| | | 20 | 68 | 36–88 | Sensorineural | | 54% | 15-96% |
| Tannahill 1979 | HHS-A and B Pre-HA Post-HA | 24 | 74 | 56–91 | Sensorineural HA users | — | 52% 10% | 14-84% 1-61% |
| Brunt 1979 | HHS- (form not reported) | 26 | 72 | 57–90 | Sensorineural | Better Poorer | 31% | 0-64% |
| Noble and Atherley 1970 | HHS | 46 | — | 35–65 | Noise-induced | — | — | — |
| McCartney et al. 1976 | HHS | 36 | 75 | 62–89 | Mostly sensorineural | Better | 70% | 19-103 |
| Kuller 1976 | HHS | 40 | 83 | 67–108 | Sensorineural | Better | 100% | 7-195 |
| Ewertsen and Birk-Nielsen 1973 | SHI (Danish) | 223 | 63 | 21–92 | 190 Impaired 25 Normal | — | NA | NA |
| Rosen 1979 | SHI (English) | 120 | — | 16–65 | — | Better | 35% | NA |
| Kuller 1976 | DSCF | 40 | 83 | 67–100 | Sensorineural | Better | 10% | 1-24 |

[  ] Threshold of synthetic sentence identification test
  * = p < .05
 ** = p < .01
  + = p < .001

TABLE 4–1 (Continued)

### CORRELATIONS OF SCALE SCORES WITH AUDIOMETRIC MEASURES

| Scale Score SD | PTA | SRT | Discrimination Score | Discrimination Material | Presentation Level | Other Correlations | Material | Other Correlations | Material |
|---|---|---|---|---|---|---|---|---|---|
| A-14.7% | 0.65** | 0.70** | −0.15 | W-22 | — | −0.24 | Rhyme test | −0.69** | SAI |
| B-15.0% | 0.38** | 0.28* | −0.13 | | | −0.04 | | −0.34* | |
| NA | NA | NA | −0.46 | Rhyme | 35 dBSL | −0.51 | Rhyme test | | |
| | | | −0.32 | test | | −0.33 | in noise S/N = 0 | | |
| 22.3% | 0.72 | [0.70] | −0.52 | PB words | PB max | −0.25 | SSI with MCR = 0 | | |
| 15.1% | 0.57** | 0.56** | −0.30** | W-22 half | 35 dBSL | −0.26** | CID | | |
| 19.9% | 0.50** | 0.57** | −0.37 | lists | | −0.46** | sentences | | |
| 13.9% | 0.49** | 0.48** | −0.12 | | | −0.09 | | | |
| 11.1% | 0.39 | 0.48 | −0.22 | | | 0.35 | | | |
| 22.2% | 0.64** | 0.57** | −0.58** | W-22 | 32 dBSL | | | | |
| 21.8% | 0.54** | 0.52** | −0.49** | | | | | | |
| | 0.60** | 0.56** | −0.54** | | | | | | |
| 18.4% | 0.62$^+$ | 0.40* | −0.44** | Campbell revised W-22 | MCL | | | | |
| 24.9% | 0.58$^+$ | 0.60$^+$ | −0.33 | Campbell revised W-22 | — | | | | |
| 27.8% | 0.73 | — | — | — | — | | | | |
| 20.4% | | | −0.20 | W-22 | 40 dBSL | | | | |
| 18.1% | NA | 0.59** | −0.73** | W-22 | 45 dBSL | | | | |
| 15.2% | NA | | | | | | | | |
| 18.6% | 0.65** | 0.53** | −0.37 | W-22 | 40 dBSL | 0.64 | SSW list EC | | |
| | 0.68** | 0.49 | −0.29 | | | 0.62 | @ 50 dBSL | | |
| — | | 0.65$^+$-SF 0.59$^+$-Left | 0.58$^+$-Left 0.57$^+$-Right | W-22 | 25 dBSL | | | | |
| 21.0% | 0.52$^+$ | 0.35* | −0.40* | Campbell revised W-22 | MCL | | | | |
| 60.7% | 0.64$^+$ | 0.65$^+$ | −0.37 | Campbell revised W-22 | — | | | | |
| NA | NA | NA | NA | NA | — | | | | |
| 23.8% | 0.58** | 0.50** | −0.33** | NU-6 | 40 dBSL | −0.35** | Audiovisual | | |
| | | | −0.37** | | MCL | | discrim. @ MCL | | |
| 7.7% | 0.37 | 0.40 | −0.39 | Campbell revised W-22 | — | | | | |

TABLE 4-2
Summary of Self-Report Instruments for Assessing Hearing Handicap

| | | | | ┌─ADMINISTRATION─┐ | |
| Instrument | Author(s) | Date | Form | Time (min.) | Items |
|---|---|---|---|---|---|
| Hearing Handicap Scale (HHS) | High et al. | 1964 | self-report questionnaire | 5 | 20 |
| Hearing Measurement Scale (HMS) | Noble and Atherley | 1970 | controlled interview | 10–40 | 42 |
| Social Hearing Handicap Index (SHI) | Ewertsen and Birk-Nielsen | 1973 | self-report questionnaire | 5 | 21 |
| Denver Scale of Communication Function | Alpiner et al. | 1974 | self-report questionnaire | 15 | 25 |
| Profile Questionnaire(s) for Rating Communication Performance | Sanders | 1975 | self-report questionnaire | 15 | 6–9 |
| Denver Scale of Communication Function for Senior Citizens (DSSC) | Zarnoch and Alpiner | 1976 | self-report questionnaire | 15 | 7 |
| Hearing Performance Inventory (HPI) Experimental Form II | Giolas et al. | 1979 | self-report questionnaire | 30–55 | 158 |
| HPI, Revised Form | Lamb et al. | 1979 | self-report questionnaire | 20 | 90 |

an instrument which would also address listening problems typically associated with persons with sensorineural hearing impairments. As a result, the HMS represents an expansion both in terms of the nature of the items included and in philosophical orientation. The questionnaire is composed of forty-two items arranged in seven subtests that cover the following areas:

1. Speech-hearing.
2. Activity for nonspeech sound.
3. Localization.
4. Reaction to handicap.
5. Speech distortion.
6. Tinnitus.
7. Personal opinion of hearing loss.

The administration of this scale is performed orally by trained interviewers. The interview approach was selected to give the respondent optimal latitude in answering the individual questions. A paper and pencil version of this scale has recently become available.[1] The hearing-impaired person's responses are scored on a five-point scale, and each item is weighted separately to increase the sensitivity of the test. The whole interview is typically taped, and more than one clinician scores the responses to enhance interjudge reliability. The original presentation of the HMS (Noble and Atherly 1970) and a more recent discussion of its modifications (Noble 1978) present in some detail the authors' research regarding the reliability and validity of the scale. Although it was originally developed for a population with noise-induced hearing impairment, the authors suggest that it can be used with most persons who acquired a hearing impairment in adulthood.

The HMS shows considerable promise. It has a broader base than the HHS, and its controlled-interview format provides an improvement over the typical unstructured interview process used by most clinicians. On the other hand, it too does not systematically probe enough different communication acts to organize a rehabilitation program of any size and scope.

### denver scale of communication function

The *Denver Scale of Communication Function* (Denver Scale) developed by Alpiner et al. (1971) has a slightly different emphasis from that of the two scales discussed earlier. The Denver Scale focuses on the attitudes or feelings of the hearing-impaired person and those with whom he or she regularly interacts. The scale is made up of twenty-five questions that are answered on a seven-point scale with *Agree* and *Disagree* at the two extremes. The questions cover four areas: family, social, vocational, and general communication. The scoring procedure incorporates the use of a handy profile chart that specifies the individual's areas of strength and weakness.

The general theme of almost all of the questions centers around the respondents' personal reactions to a set of limited but representative situations. That is, the Denver Scale gives respondents the task of rating their *personal reactions* to given situations, as opposed to other scales, which ask respondents to rate how they would *perform* in that same situation. To compensate for this, Alpiner (1978) recommends the use of a supplementary scale developed by Sanders (1980) to obtain information regarding individual performance in specific communication situations.

Before discussing the profile questionnaires developed by Sanders, it is important to state that the use of an instrument such as the Denver Scale to assess aural rehabilitation programs, hearing aid candidacy, and successful hearing aid use and to generate a profile of attitudes toward communicative performance is certainly a step in the right direction. Used creatively,

---

[1]Copies of both versions of the Hearing Measurement Scale may be obtained by writing to The University of New England Publishing Unit, The University of New England, Armidale, N.S.W. 2351, Australia.

the Denver Scale can be a valuable clinical tool. It is reliable (McNeill and Alpiner 1975) and touches on extremely relevant issues in a hearing-impaired person's life. Furthermore, the Denver Scale appeared when nothing of its kind was available and, like the Hearing Handicap Scale, it expanded the concept of assessing the handicapping effects of hearing impairment. A copy of the Denver Scale can be found in Appendix D.

### profile questionnaires for rating communicative performance

Sanders (1980) recognized the need to expand clinical information for aural rehabilitation beyond the personal reaction data generated by the Denver Scale. He proposed profile questionnaires, an interesting format by which clinicians can develop their own set of questions tailored specifically to the particular person for whom aural rehabilitation is being considered. He suggests that the questions center around three basic communication settings: home, business, and social environments.

This individualized approach has merit and will appeal to some clinicians. A unique contribution made by this approach lies in its scoring procedure. The questions are answered in two parts: degree of difficulty on a scale from +2 to –2, and frequency of occurrence on a scale from 1 to 3. The product of these two numbers provides information which incorporates the value of the question as well as of the answer and is a reflection of the importance of the specific situation for that individual.

### section summary

A number of instruments have been developed to assess hearing handicap. Four of these procedures which have played an important role in generating interest in the self-report approach were discussed. Each of these procedures has its unique orientation, and when the procedures are combined with one another and with audiological data, they will most likely generate meaningful information for rehabilitation purposes. However, review of these procedures has revealed that no single instrument has sufficient scope in terms of a variety of listening situations nor does it contain a large enough corpus of questions to provide the desired comprehensive description necessary to plan a tailor-made rehabilitation program. It was this conclusion that led to the development of the Hearing Performance Inventory (Giolas, Owens, Lamb, and Schubert 1979).

### hearing performance inventory

The Hearing Performance Inventory (HPI) was developed to provide a systematic procedure for identifying the variety of problem areas experienced by persons as a result of their hearing impairment. The overall goal was to create a measuring instrument with sufficient scope to yield a profile of hearing performance in a variety of everyday listening situations. The obtained profiles could be used to organize rehabilitation programs, plan initial rehabilitation activities, and suggest a more meaningful progression of management activities, thereby supplementing the customary audiology report. To achieve the comprehensiveness desired and to yield specific rehabilitation objectives, the inventory items were divided into six sections entitled: (1) *Understanding Speech;* (2) *Intensity;* (3) *Response to Auditory Failure;* (4) *Social;* (5) *Personal;* and (6) *Occupational.* It is hoped that such an inventory will provide:

1. An indication of whether the hearing impairment has manifested itself as a communication problem.
2. A detailed analysis of the communication breakdown, allowing a tailor-made management program to emerge sooner than is now possible.
3. A quantitative measure of performance both for initial assessment and for evidence of progress.

***The Basic Format.*** The basic format of the HPI consists of presenting the hearing-impaired person with a set of everyday listening situations and asking for a judgment on how the person performs in these situations. For example, one item of the inventory reads: "You are with a male friend or family member in a fairly quiet room. Can you understand him when his voice is loud enough for you and you can see his face?"

The hearing-impaired person is asked to judge how often he or she experiences difficulty in each designated situation and to respond using the following categories: *Practically always; Frequently; About half the time; Occasionally;* and *Almost never.* For scoring and for computing statistical summaries, numbers 1 to 5 are assigned to these five descriptive responses. According to Simpson (1963), the quantitative meaning of these verbal descriptions corresponded to approximately 100%, 75%, 50%, 25% and 0%, respectively. If the situation described is not in the person's experience repertoire then the item *Does not apply* should be marked.

The self-report approach was selected because the developers of the HPI were convinced that aural rehabilitation programs must take into account early the person's own perceived areas of difficulty if management is to be meaningful and motivating. The accuracy of the individuals' judgments regarding the effects of their hearing impairments on their everyday life situations is not assumed. In the absence of validity criteria, the judgments are used as a starting point for rehabilitation, mindful of the findings of Silverman et al. (1948). These investigators concluded that answers from hearing-impaired persons reflected too heavily their attitudes toward the difficulty rather than the actual magnitude of the communication problem. These two aspects must be explored separately to ascertain which rehabilitative measures are needed. The use of the self-report procedure in this context requires that the respondent's judgments be checked against (1) the ever-increasing information gained through standard audiological data; (2) a critical informant's (e.g., spouse's) perceptions of the hearing-impaired person's listening performance; and, of course, (3) the clinician's own observations. Taking into account these qualifying factors, the rationale for using the self-report approach is twofold:

1. There is rehabilitative value in assessing hearing-impaired persons' perceptions of their performance in listening situations which comprise their overall personal communication setting.

2. In the clinical setting, the accuracy of these perceptions is less important initially in that they are used as a starting point for selecting rehabilitative activities, with accuracy checks emerging as management progresses.

The question of the validity of any measure attempting to assess handicap can always be raised. The complexity of human behavior is such that cause-and-effect information of the type that is necessary when measuring the effect of hearing impairment on human behavior is almost impossible to demonstrate. On the other hand, such validity is not a necessary prerequisite to the use of self-report instruments in this context. The goal is to obtain information about the kinds of problems a particular person perceives that he or she is experiencing. To accomplish this, items must be representative of typical problems experienced by hearing-impaired persons in general, and there must be good test-retest reliability. In this way, reliable information about a particular person's perceptions can be ascertained in order to evolve a personalized rehabilitative program. When measuring progress, hearing-impaired persons can be used as their own controls. This, of course, assumes a cooperative and sincere respondent who will be seen in a clinical setting over time as part of an overall rehabilitation program. Assessing handicap for other purposes, such as compensation for disability on a one-shot basis, is considerably more complex and may well require a completely different approach.

Finally, it should be noted that the developers of the HPI chose to use the term *performance* rather than *handicap* in naming their inventory. This is consistent with this writer's contention that the instrument is simply measuring the respondents' perceptions of how they perform in the listening situations described. Whether these perceptions are real and to what degree they manifest a handicap is not known at this time. This still remains a challenge to the clinician.

The HPI has gone through three major revisions. Each revision will be discussed separately. The revisions were undertaken in the interest of rendering the inventory clinically practical while at the same time maintaining its comprehensive nature.

***Experimental Form I.***   Initially, each investigator generated as many items as possible describing a multitude of consequences resulting from having a hearing impairment. Over 500 possible items resulted, oriented toward a number of areas of communication difficulty. Next, extended discussion by the investigators narrowed the selection to a prototype set of 289 items. Decisions about retaining or discarding any of these still-untested items were influenced by input from:

1. Hearing-impaired persons.
2. Audiologists, including two with hearing impairment.
3. Normally hearing persons.
4. A study conducted by Nett et al. (1960) which assessed a number of hard-of-hearing adults in a variety of ways and described them in terms of reported communication problems.

The set of 289 items, constituting the first experimental form, was administered to 220 hearing-impaired persons. The only requirement for participation was an expression of communicative difficulty secondary to hearing loss. Most of the respondents were enrolled in rehabilitation programs or completed the inventory during the course of a clinic visit for an audiologic evaluation that had revealed a hearing loss. For this sample, no attempt was made to collect complete audiological data on all participants.

A total of 220 respondents completed the 289-item inventory. They were all urged to comment on the items. Of the 220 forms, 190 were sufficiently complete for item analysis. The statistical measures included a mean, a median, a mean rank, a standard deviation, a standard error of the mean for each item, and a histogram (i.e., a breakdown of the number of subjects who selected each of the five responses). When items differed on only one dimension (e.g., male versus female, noises versus quiet), a .20 or larger difference in standard error was taken as an indication of a statistically significant difference between item means (P < .05). When there was no significant difference, either the items were combined or the preferred one was retained. In other instances items were eliminated on the basis of: (1) badly skewed distributions (too many 1 or 5 responses); (2) narrow distribution of responses; (3) a large proportion of omissions; (4) inappropriateness as judged by a high proportion of the respondents. Occasionally an otherwise-marginal item was retained because of its relevance to a specific goal of rehabilitation. On the basis of statistical performance and respondent reports, over half of the items were retained, sometimes with modifications in wording.

Based on this critical item evaluation, several useful observations emerged and a number of changes were made. A summary of these observations may be found in Appendix E.

Some additional descriptive statistics are of interest. The average item score (mean) was 2.6, approximately halfway between the response extremes of *Almost never* and *Practically always;* the average item standard deviation was 1.2. The distribution of responses is shown in Figure 4–1. It should be remembered that this description may change with further sampling. For example, many of the items with a high concentration of 1 responses *(No difficulty)* were eliminated, so that the remaining items will generate an average response which will migrate toward 3. The items retained constitute Experimental Form II.

***Experimental Form II.*** The second revision of the inventory (Form II) consists of 158 items and can be administered in approximately forty-five minutes. The 27 occupational items are placed at the end and can be conveniently omitted by respondents who are not employed, resulting in a further saving of time. The six sections, which were listed earlier, assess most common listening situations with different speakers in different communication situations and different noise environments. Each section will be discussed separately.

Table 4–3 outlines the categories and subcategories assessed in the section entitled *Understanding Speech.* As can be seen, an attempt is made by this section to assess a variety of parameters representative of everyday conversational situations. This particular section represents the kinds of problems a hearing-impaired person might have with speech discrimination. The respondent is asked to judge how well he or she can understand what people are saying when their voices are loud enough. In the instructions the term *understand* is operationally defined as hearing the words of a speaker clearly

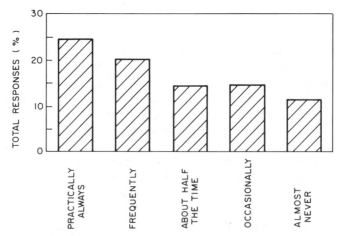

FIGURE 4–1 Distribution of Responses for the Approximately 200 Respondents Who Filled Out Experimental Form 1. (Giolas et al. 1979)

TABLE 4-3
Categories and Subcategories in the *Understanding Speech* Section

Each set of ( ) and [ ] contains number of items in each grouping. Items from the *Social* section are included. The first entry in each ( ) or [ ] indicates the number of items with visual cues; the second entry indicates the number of items with no visual cues. See Appendix F for identification of specific items. ( ) refer to Experimental Form II; [ ] refer to Revised Form.

| Talker | Communicative Situation | Communication System | Noise Environment |
|---|---|---|---|
| Male (9, 2); [3, 4] | One-to-one* (alone) (15, 16); [7, 2] | Telephone (0, 2); [0, 1] | Fairly quiet (14, 10); [7, 6] |
| Female (10, 2); [6, 1] | One-to-one** (group) (9, 4); [5, 1] | Television (4, 0); [3, 0] | Music, etc. (16, 10); [9, 4] |
| | Group conversation (10, 10)**; [5, 6] | Play or movie (2, 0); [1, 0] | People talking nearby (12, 0); [5, 0] |
| Child (3, 0); [2, 0] | 5 or 6 friends/family members (5, 4); [1, 2] | Public address (2, 2); [1, 1] | |
| Friend/family members (16, 4); [7, 2] | 5 or 6 strangers (3, 2); [3, 1] | Auditorium (2, 1); [1, 0] | |
| Stranger (5, 3); [3, 1] | 1 talker at a time (6, 5); [3, 3] | Bus, air depot (0, 1); [0, 1] | |
| | Aware of subject (3, 4); [1, 2] | | |
| Waiter/waitress (3, 0); [2, 0] | Subject changes (3, 3); [2, 1] | | |
| | Talkers interrupting (1, 0); [1, 0] | | |
| | Automobile (2, 2); [1, 2] | | |
| | Games (0, 2); [0, 1] | | |

*In one-to-one situations the talker is speaking directly to the respondent, whether in a group or a 2-person situation. Inclusion of waiter/waitress items may be debatable.

**Items of the subheadings under *Group conversation* are not mutually exclusive and thus do not equal the total.

Giolas et al., 1979.

enough to be able to participate in the conversation. In a number of items there are no visual cues to understanding because the speaker's face is not visible. Below are listed three examples of questions appearing in this section.

1. You are in a fairly quiet room. Can you carry on a conversation with a woman in another room if her voice is loud enough for you?

2. You are with a male friend or family member and several people are talking nearby. Can you understand him when his voice is loud enough for you and you can see his face?

63

3. You are at a party or gathering of more than twenty people and there is background noise such as music or a crowd of people. Can you understand what a stranger is saying to you when his/her voice is loud enough for you and you can see his/her face?

Table 4–4 outlines the categories and subcategories assessed in the section entitled *Intensity*. One of the primary factors determining level of performance in many listening situations is the degree of the hearing loss. The items included in this section represent a number of listening tasks. Respondents judge whether they are aware of designated auditory stimuli in different situations. The items in this section ask the respondents to judge only how often they are aware of the occurrence of a particular sound (e.g., doorbell, speech). Below are listed three examples of questions appearing in this section.

1. If you are riding in a car and you know that others are listening to music on the car radio, do you hear the music?
2. How often do men speak loudly enough for you to hear them?
3. You are in a fairly quiet room and a person is talking to you from a distance of no more than six feet. Would you be aware that he/she is talking if you did not see his/her face?

It is important to assess not only areas of difficulty experienced in typical listening situations but also what is done to compensate for this difficulty.

TABLE 4–4
Categories and Subcategories in the *Intensity* Section

( )/[ ] indicate number of items. See Appendix F for specific items. ( ) refer to Experimental Form II; [ ] refer to Revised Form.

| Talker | Communicative Situation | Communication System | Nonspeech Stimuli | Noise Environment |
|---|---|---|---|---|
| Male (1); [0] | One-to one (5); [3] | Public address (1); [1] | Doorbell (2); [1] | Fairly quiet (4); [1] |
| Female (1); [0] | Other room (2); [1] | Radio or TV (2); [1] | Telephone ringing (2); [0] | Music, etc. (5); [3] |
| Child (1); [1] | 6 feet away (2); [1] | | Refrigerator (1); [0] | |
| | Whisper (1); [1] | | Water running (1); [1] | |
| | | | Birds singing (1); [0] | |
| | | | Airplane (1); [1] | |
| | | | Music (car radio) (1); [0] | |

Giolas et al., 1979.

Consequently, a section entitled *Response to Auditory Failure* was developed, as shown in Table 4–5. The items in this section ask the respondent how frequently he or she uses a particular behavior (e.g., asking for repetition, adjusting hearing aid) in the designated listening situation. This section incidentally directs the respondent's attention to behavior which may enhance or detract from his or her communicative efficiency. The following two questions are examples of the questions appearing in this section.

1. You are talking with a close friend. When you miss something important that was said, do you immediately adjust your hearing aid to help you hear better?

2. You are with five or six friends or family members. One person talks at a time. When you miss something important that was said, do you pretend you understood?

The social effects of the hearing impairment are assessed by items describing a number of conversational situations stressing social interaction outside of occupational settings. The *Social* section of the inventory is derived from selected items in the *Understanding Speech* and *Response to Auditory Failure* sections. Categories and subcategories are shown in Table 4–6. To be included in the *Social* section, an item had to involve a group of more than two persons convened primarily for recreation, which is broadly de-

TABLE 4–5
Categories and Subcategories in the *Response to Auditory Failure* Section

( ) refer to Experimental Form II; [ ] refer to Revised Form. See Appendix F for identification of specific items.

| Talker | Communicative Situation | Behavior Assessed |
|---|---|---|
| Friend/family member (4); [3] | One-to-one (8); [5] | Adjust hearing aid (2); [1] |
| Stranger (3); [1] | Group conversation (8); [4] | Ask for assistance or favor (6); [4] |
| Waiter/waitress (2); [1] | 1 talker at a time (4); [1] | Ask for repetition (7); [5] |
| | Talkers interrupting (4); [3] | Ask for repeat of portion* (5); [3] |
| | Social situations (18); [12] | Inform of loss (6); [2] |
| | | Keep trying (1); [0] |
| | | Move seat (3); [2] |
| | | Pretend to understand (3); [3] |

*Refers to practice of asking for only part of message not understood. We call this selective questioning.
Giolas et al., 1979.

TABLE 4–6
Categories and Subcategories in the *Social* Section

Items from *Understanding Speech* (with visual cues and with no visual cues) and *Response to Auditory Failure* are included. ( ) refer to Experimental Form II; [ ] refer to Revised Form.

| Talkers | Communicative Situation | Behavior Assessed | Noise Environment |
|---|---|---|---|
| Male (2); [1] | One-to-one (group) (13); [6] | Adjust hearing aid (1); [0] | Fairly quiet (10); [2] |
| Female (2); [1] | Group conversation (37); [21] | Ask for assistance or favor (2); [0] | Music, etc. (15); [4] |
| Friend/family member (11); [5] | 5 or 6 friends/family members (19); [9] | Ask for repetition (4); [4] | People talking nearby (7); [3] |
| Stranger (2); [1] | 5 or 6 strangers (11); [7] | Ask for repeat of portion (3); [1] | |
| | 1 talker at a time (15); [7] | Inform of loss (4); [2] | |
| | Aware of subject (7); [3] | Move seat (2); [1] | |
| | Subject changes (6); [3] | Pretend to understand (2); [2] | |
| | Talkers interrupting (5); [4] | | |
| | Automobile (4); [3] | | |
| | Games (2); [1] | | |
| | Small gathering (1); [1] | | |
| | Dinner (4); [2] | | |

Giolas et al., 1979.

fined to include dining, conversing, playing games, etc. The following is an example of a question appearing in this section.

1. You are at a party or gathering of less than ten people and the room is fairly quiet. Can you understand what a friend or family member is saying to you when his/her voice is loud enough for you and you can see his/her face?

Eight items constituting the *Personal* section deal primarily with how the respondents feel about their hearing impairment as it influences their self-esteem and social interaction. A table or other breakdown for these items does not seem warranted because they occur sequentially in the inventory and may be appraised at a glance. Below are listed four examples of questions appearing in this section.

1. Does your hearing problem discourage you from going to the movies?
2. Does your hearing problem lower your self-confidence?
3. Does your hearing problem tend to make you impatient?
4. Do you feel that others cannot understand what it is to have a hearing problem?

Finally, the items constituting the *Occupational* section explore some of the dimensions of hearing impairment within an occupational context, as shown in Table 4–7. This section may be given to persons currently employed and also to those recently employed or those participating in activities similar to employment, such as attending school or doing volunteer work. The following question appears in this section.

1. You are in a fairly quiet room at work with five or six coworkers. One person talks at a time. When you are aware of the subject, can you understand what is being said when the speaker's voice is loud enough for you and you can see his/her face?

The specific items, by number, constituting all of the sections, categories, and subcategories of the HPI are shown in Appendix F. The *Social* and *Occupational* items are included with the *Understanding Speech* and *Response to*

TABLE 4–7
Categories and Subcategories in the *Occupational* Section

Items from *Understanding Speech* and *Response to Auditory Failure* are included. ( ) refer to Experimental Form II; [ ] refer to Revised Form.

| Talker | Communicative Situation | Behavior Assessed | Noise Environment |
|---|---|---|---|
| Male (3); [2] | One-to one (18); [10] | Adjust hearing aid (2); [2] | Fairly quiet (5); [3] |
| Female (3); [2] | Group conversation (6); [3] | Ask for repetition (1); [1] | Music, etc. (3); [2] |
| Coworker (12); [9] | 5 or 6 coworkers (6); [2] | Ask for repeat of portion (2); [1] | People talking nearby (7); [1] |
| Employer (7); [2] | 1 talker at a time (5); [2] | Inform of loss (3); [1] | |
| | Talkers interrupting (1); [1] | Pretend to understand (3); [2] | |
| | Aware of subject (1) | | |
| | Subject changes (2); [1] | | |

Giolas et al., 1979.

*Auditory Failure* sections. *Understanding Speech* items with no visual cues are treated as a separate entity in the item listing.

**Revised Form.** The third and most recent revision of the HPI was designed to refine the HPI so that it could be administered within a shorter time interval without sacrificing any of the specific clinical objectives. It consists of a total of 90 items and has not eliminated any of the original sections or crucial categories. The *Occupational* section has been reduced to 15 items and again appears at the end of the Inventory for convenient elimination if desired. The remaining items have been randomized throughout the Inventory. The shortened version has reduced the administration time to approximately twenty minutes. No significant changes have been made in the test administration or scoring procedures. A breakdown of items by section, category, and subcategory may be found in Tables 4–3, 4–4, 4–5, 4–6, 4–7 and Appendix G. A copy of the entire Revised Form may also be found in Appendix G.

At the present time it appears that the revised version of the HPI can be used in most clinical settings. It is sufficiently comprehensive in scope (number of items) to yield rehabilitative clues yet takes considerably less time to administer and score than the earlier version. However, as rehabilitation progresses, the need to further assess performance in everyday listening situations may arise. The longer form will provide the additional pool of items. Furthermore, the longer version may lend itself to the more detailed analysis often desired in research settings.

**Clinical Administration.** The hearing-impaired person is presented with the Inventory, an answer sheet, and a set of instructions (see Appendix F), which are read aloud by the clinician as each individual follows on a separate copy. Special care should be taken to explain the five-choice response system, the talker reference, and terms such as *aware, hear,* and *understand.* The individual is encouraged to ask questions about the procedure, and two or three items are worked through with each person. Also, it is best if the clinician is available for questions throughout the procedure. Frequently the respondents inquire about a specific item and must be encouraged to answer according to the way they behave most often or according to the way most people talk to them.

It should be remembered that the five descriptive responses for each item are assigned numerical values of 1 to 5. In the scoring process, an overall percentage of difficulty may be obtained by adding the numerical responses for all items attempted, dividing by the number of items attempted, and multiplying by 20. (Items with *Does not apply* responses as well as omitted items are counted as not attempted.) A comparable procedure may be followed for each section and, if desired, for categories within or cutting across sections when there are sufficient items for meaningful appraisal.

Because the respondent is asked to judge an item on a scale from 1 to 5 with 5 suggesting maximum difficulty, the above scoring procedure will yield a score of 20% (the minimum obtainable) for little or no difficulty and a score of 100% for maximum difficulty. In this connection, the most natural wording for *Personal* items and *Response to Auditory Failure* items dealing with pretending to understand requires that the responses be reversed: that is, 1 corresponds to least appropriate behavior and 5 to most appropriate behavior, in contrast to other items of the inventory. Therefore, these items must be flagged and the response numbers must be reversed (a 1 becomes a 5 and a 4 becomes a 2) before proceeding with the scoring.

***Clinical Application.***   At the present time, the HPI is not seen as an integral part of the standard battery of audiological tests administered at the initial visit. The primary purpose of the initial visit is to assess the presence and nature of the possible hearing impairment. It appears to have its greatest utility in describing the adverse effect of the hearing impairment on the person's everyday life and in assisting the clinician in planning and assessing the effectiveness of nonmedical rehabilitative procedures such as amplification and communication skills classes. In these instances, and using Experimental Form II, this writer generates a performance profile for the following five section scores: (1) *Understanding speech,* (2) *Intensity,* (3) *Response to auditory failure,* (4) *Social,* and, when appropriate, (5) *Occupational.* (The *Personal* section is not typically included because there are so few items comprising the section.) A typical profile generated for section scores is shown in Figure 4–2. The items comprising each section are listed in Appendix F under *Sections.* Using the same verbal markers supplied by the respondent—*practically always* (100%), *frequently* (75%), *about half the time* (50%), *occasionally* (25%), and *almost never* (0%)—the profile suggests that the respondent reports *having difficulty about half the time (scores vary between 40% and 50%)* in all the communicative situations assessed.

Depending on the hearing-impaired person's responses, expanded profiles can be plotted for selected categories within various sections. For most persons, a section profile for the *Understanding Speech, Social* and *Response to Auditory Failure* will prove most helpful. The items comprising the profile headings are listed in Appendix F under *Categories and Subcategories.* The profile headings are derived from the table headings for each section presented earlier in this chapter. The reader may want to consult these tables and select his or her own profile headings. Appendix F is organized to parallel the section tables to facilitate generation of new profile headings. The following guidelines are offered to facilitate identifying the items comprising the Understanding Speech and Social profiles presented in this chapter. The remaining profiles are self-explanatory.

1. The items used to generate scores for the categories of Talker and Communicative Situations include items in both the Visual and Nonvisual Cues categories.

2. The items used to generate scores for the One-to-one group subcategory include all items listed under (1) One-to-one group < 10, (2) One-to-one in group > 20; and (3) One-to-one in group playing cards, etc.

3. The items used to generate scores for the subcategory of Group Conversations include all items listed in the One-to-one group (number 2 above) as well as those items listed under Group Conversations.

4. Social items are underlined and Occupational items are in parentheses and are found in Appendix F in the Understanding Speech and Response to Auditory Failure sections.

Figures 4–3, 4–4, and 4–5 illustrate typical profiles plotted for these sections. By inspection of these profiles, the following statements can be made:

*Understanding Speech* (Figure 4–3) The respondent reports:

1. difficulty (occasionally—40-46%) in communicative situations where there are unfamiliar speakers, group conversations, public address systems, and noise in the background (music, etc.) and when there are interruptions (more than half the time—60%).

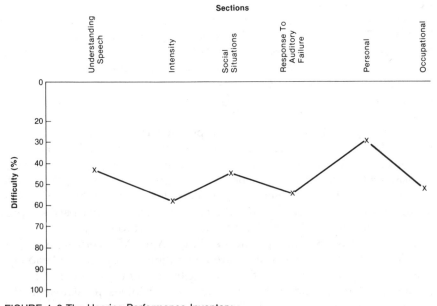

FIGURE 4–2 The Hearing Performance Inventory

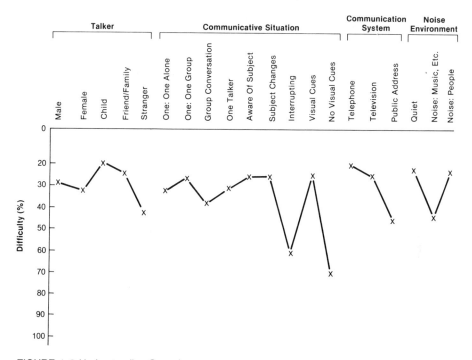

UNDERSTANDING SPEECH

FIGURE 4–3 Understanding Speech

*Social* (Figure 4–4) The respondent reports:

1. having more difficulty understanding speech in social situations when the speaker is a stranger (more than half the time—60%) but practically always (20%) understands when the speaker is a friend or family member.

2. understanding speech in quiet (20%) social situations but as often as not (52%) experiences difficulty in noise situations which involve background music, etc.

*Response to Auditory Failure* (Figure 4–5) The respondent reports:

1. frequently asking for a repetition (37%) or repeating a portion of what was heard (36%), as often as not asking for assistance (67%) or pretending to have understood (60%). The respondent never informs the speaker about the hearing impairment (100%).

2. employing the behaviors assessed in the Response to Auditory Failure section frequently (40%) with friends and family members and only occasionally (80%) with strangers.

For purposes of discussion with the respondent, it is often helpful to generate a performance profile for the *Intensity* section. The profile shown

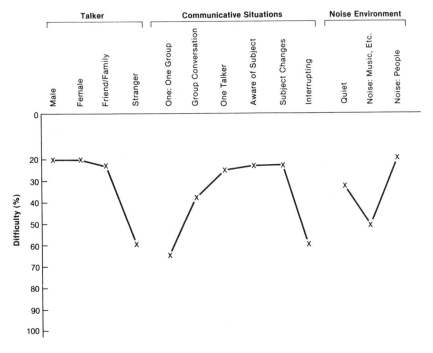

FIGURE 4–4 Social

in Figure 4–6 indicates that the respondent reports *only occasionally (80%)* *hearing stimuli from the other room or in a noisy environment.*

When the respondent is employed, a profile can be plotted for the *Occupational* section (see Figure 4–7). By inspection of this profile, it can be seen that in the occupational setting the respondent reports *difficulty understanding employer and coworkers occasionally (30-40%), more so in group conversations (40%) and when others are interrupting the conversation (60%).*

The HPI percentage scores, depicted in profiles, offer a convenient manner of organizing the respondents' judgments of their performance in everyday listening situations. Once profile headings are determined, the scoring process can be greatly facilitated through the use of templates. For example, respondents are asked to record their answers on a standard answer sheet which contains all item responses on two sides of one sheet (available at no cost through Prentice-Hall; see Appendix F). Templates are then made to fit the answer sheet and provide a quick way in which to identify the items comprising each of the five HPI sections and a section profile (Figure 4–2) is plotted. Templates may also be made to facilitate identifying the items

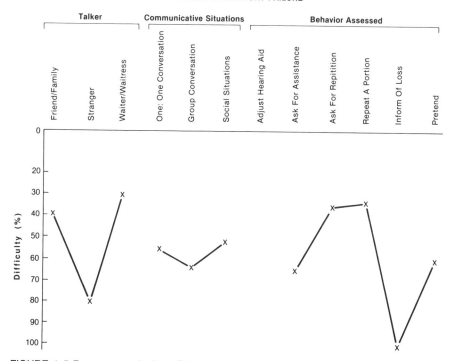

FIGURE 4–5 Response to Auditory Failure

comprising the categories and subcategories of the expanded profiles for each section, e.g., Figures 4–3 through 4–7.*

Bevan (1977) in some preliminary work has demonstrated that useful profiles can be generated and that they differ from person to person. After reviewing these profiles with the respondent, the clinician can make decisions jointly with the respondent regarding areas which need to be worked on immediately and areas which need further exploration. A more extensive discussion on how the HPI can be linked with management planning will follow in Chapter Five.

*Normal Listeners and HPI.* Chasser (1978) and Chasser and Giolas (1977) conducted a pilot study designed to examine the performance of normally hearing adults on the HPI. It was hypothesized that this population would experience minimal difficulty in the listening situations described. These findings might provide a baseline for comparison between

*Templates for several categories of the Revised Form are available through Dr. S. Lamb, San Francisco State University, San Francisco, Ca.

INTENSITY

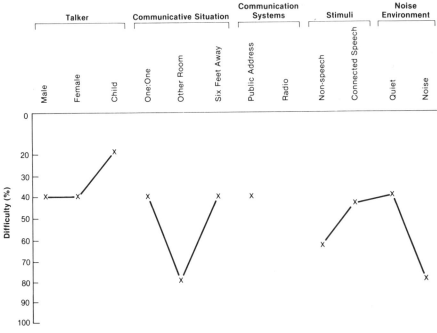

FIGURE 4–6 Intensity

the performance of normally hearing and hearing-impaired adults on the HPI. The question of test-retest reliability was also addressed with this population.

The group of subjects consisted of twenty-five normally hearing adults (eight males and seventeen females) between the ages of 25 and 55 years with a mean age of 37.6. The HPI was administered individually two times eight to ten weeks apart. Mean percentage scores and standard deviations were computed for five sections of the HPI (*Personal* was omitted) and for categories within each section.

Mean scores for all sections assessed are presented in Table 4–8. As can be seen, persons with normal hearing report little difficulty in listening situations described in the *Understanding Speech, Intensity,* and *Social* sections. The mean percent scores obtained for these sections correlate to mean response scores centering around *Practically always* and *Frequently* in terms of how often the respondents believe they perform well in these situations. Figure 4-8 plots a profile of the mean percentage scores for these sections.

The mean percentage score for the *Response to Auditory Failure* section is of particular interest. This section deals exclusively with what a person does when confronted with a difficult listening situation. The less often the respondent reports using the strategies assessed, the higher the percentage

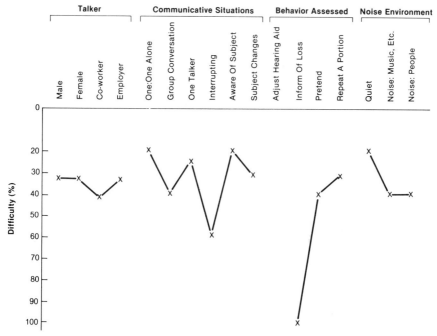

FIGURE 4-7 Occupational

score. The overall mean of 68.8% and standard deviation of 16.9 obtained for this section suggest that the normally hearing subjects employ the strategies assessed about half the time and that there is considerable variability in their responses. The variability is probably due to the fact that normally hearing persons do not routinely miss what is being said and, consequently, do not develop an elaborate set of strategies to handle such occasions when they arise.

This information about normally hearing persons seems to have great importance for dealing appropriately with the hearing-impaired population. If a hearing-impaired person does not get appropriate counseling and other

TABLE 4-8
Subtest Means and Standard Deviations for
Normal Hearing Subjects on the HPI

| Section | Mean | Standard Deviation |
|---|---|---|
| Understanding Speech | 1.56 | .27 |
| Intensity | 1.13 | .14 |
| Response to Auditory Failure | 3.28 | .56 |
| Social | 2.43 | .38 |
| Occupational | 1.70 | 1.00 |

From Chasser 1977.

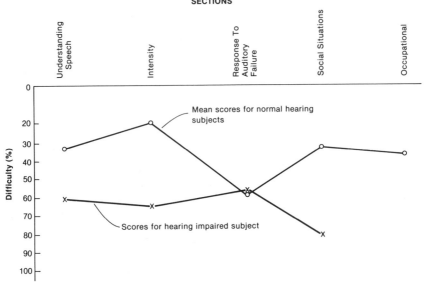

THE HEARING PERFORMANCE INVENTORY
SECTIONS

FIGURE 4–8 The Hearing Performance Inventory. (Data from C. Chasser 1977)

treatment in an aural rehabilitation program, he or she may respond to auditory failure in the same manner as the normally hearing person. If a hearing-impaired person obtains a score that corresponds to that of a normally hearing person, it is essential for the clinician to incorporate appropriate responses to auditory failure into an aural rehabilitation program.

Chasser (1977) also examined the test-retest reliability of the HPI with normally hearing adults. He computed a Pearson Product Moment Correlation Coefficient by finding the square root of the average coefficient of determination for each item. A correlation coefficient of .74 was obtained, which was considered good in that (1) the proportion of subjects compared to total test items was small, (2) the five-point scale limits reliability, and (3) lower test-retest correlations are typically obtained for paper-and-pencil tests of this kind. This correlation, which explains approximately 50% of the variance from one test setting to another, is encouraging.

This chapter presented a rationale for assessing the handicapping effect of hearing impairment through the use of a self-report approach. Some of the reasons for the recent interest in this approach were outlined and some of the more frequently used and recently developed instruments were discussed. These instruments include the Hearing Handicap Scale, the Hearing Measurement Scale, the Denver Scale of Communication Function, the Profile Questionnaires for Rating Communicative Performance, and the Hearing Performance Inventory. Special emphasis was placed on the Hearing Performance Inventory in terms of its development and clinical implications for planning aural rehabilitation programs. It was pointed out that two of the major responsibilities of clinical audiologists are: (1) assessing the handicapping effects of hearing impairment, especially in terms of communication, and (2) gauging the success of any rehabilitative process (medical or nonmedical) in terms of the alleviation or minimizing of these handicapping effects. The audiologist was urged to consider the use of the self-report procedure to execute this responsibility.

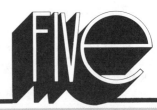

# Aural rehabilitation: an orientation

The last decade has seen increased interest in rehabilitative programs for persons who have acquired hearing impairments as adults. These programs have changed considerably from the lipreading classes of the early years. They have expanded their goals to include a broader approach to the communication process. In 1974 the Committee on Rehabilitative Audiology of the American Speech-Lanugage-Hearing Association (ASHA) outlined the basic components of a contemporary program as follows:

1. Selection of an amplification system to make available as much undistorted sensory information as possible.
2. Development, remediation, or conservation of receptive and expressive language abilities.
3. Counseling for client and family.
4. Continuing reevaluation of auditory function.
5. Assessment of the effectiveness of rehabilitative procedures.

Regardless of the unique orientations and differences in specific activities comprising the numerous programs described in the literature, they all appear to share a common goal, which is to help hearing-impaired persons develop their optimal potential in communication (ASHA 1974). While these programs are too numerous and overlapping to describe here, the reader is referred to Fleming (1972) and Hardick (1977) for concise descriptions of two representative orientations to aural rehabilitation.

The purpose of this chapter is to discuss the essentials of a comprehensive aural rehabilitation program. These essentials will be discussed in general terms so as to allow for their adaptation to different professional settings and to allow for the individual preferences of the clinicians involved. In deference to tradition, the term *aural rehabilitation* will be used, as opposed to *audiologic habilitation,* the term suggested by ASHA (1974). As the discussion unfolds, it may occur to some readers that the term *hearing conservation* would be the more appropriate term to use for the comprehensive program being described. While in many ways it is a term preferred by this writer, once again we are bowing to tradition and avoiding it to minimize any confusion with the very important and specific hearing conservation programs being conducted in industry and the public schools.

## ○ A COMPREHENSIVE AURAL REHABILITATION PROGRAM

There is probably no single rehabilitative process in the area of communication disorders that has been more misunderstood than aural rehabilitation. It has been viewed as a series of lipreading classes or, in more recent years, it has been expanded to include the use of visual cues in general. It has been described as consisting solely of the hearing aid evaluation and orientation process. Along these lines, another approach is to put amplification into the broader context of auditory training and to extend aural rehabilitation to include activities designed to facilitate the optimal use of residual hearing. The aural rehabilitation process is viewed by some as centering on providing basic information about hearing impairment and its effect on communication. Finally, there is the self-help approach to aural rehabilitation. It focuses primarily, through various philosophical orientations, on what people can do to help themselves in difficult listening situations.

Aural rehabilitation contains all these components and more. When it is viewed narrowly as encompassing one or two or even three of these components, it does a partial job at best and fails miserably at worst.

It follows, therefore, that an aural rehabilitation program must be designed so that it meets the comprehensive service needs of the target population. The central concern of the services should be verbal communication. However, ways in which a breakdown in the communication process impacts on other everyday activities should also be of concern and should be dealt with directly or indirectly through referral. The following sections will outline a comprehensive aural rehabilitation program. The degree to which the audiologist is directly or indirectly involved will also be noted, and suggestions regarding referrals to appropriate disciplines will be included.

## ○ PUBLIC INFORMATION AND AUDIOMETRIC SCREENING

One of the most important functions of a comprehensive aural rehabilitation program is informing the public about the nature of hearing impairment and its handicapping effects. Given that the progression of this disorder is often gradual (as in presbycusis) and that there is frequently resistance to accepting the reality of reduced hearing, the public must be provided with an opportunity to learn about the potential ramifications of hearing impairment. Furthermore, hopefully this information will come along at a time when hearing-impaired persons are just beginning to suspect that everyone else does not really mumble or talk too softly or make too much background noise but that the problem may lie in their own inability to hear normally.

These public information programs must take a very different approach from that of the many advertisements and magazine articles that associate hearing impairment exclusively with hearing aids. When first confronted with a hearing problem, few people are ready for a hearing aid. They are eager, however, for information which will help them understand what they are experiencing. Such information can be provided by conducting a series of lectures and discussion groups in the community (e.g., through social organizations or senior citizen groups) which center around hearing in general and which present the material at an elementary and practical level. The goal is to alert the public to the numerous reasons for faulty hearing. Discussions may include subjects such as hearing and its disorders, the need for medical consultation, good listening habits, communication strategies to use when auditory failures occur, and the effect of poor environmental conditions. These discussions should be designed to motivate hearing-impaired persons to seek professional help if they are experiencing difficulty.

The audience need not be restricted to persons with known or suspected hearing impairment. In fact, all interested persons should be encouraged to attend. In that way, the personal threat often felt by persons who suspect they have hearing impairment is reduced, and spouses and close friends can gain a better understanding of the manifestations of hearing impairment.

The topics should be quite general and designed to stimulate discussion. It is a good idea for the audiologist to remain for a brief period following the program so that persons wishing to ask individual questions will have that opportunity.

Audiometric screening may also be included as part of a public information program. If this is done, the purpose is to test those persons wishing to learn more about their hearing. The results should be briefly discussed with each person, and appropriate referrals should be made (Hardick 1977). Caution should be taken to avoid presenting the audiometric screening as the main purpose of the program. This would give the program the image of being only for persons with acknowledged hearing impairment, and thus a very important segment of the target population would be lost.

As these lectures progress, one or two persons may start mentioning their own hearing difficulties or may bring in an old unused hearing aid of theirs or their spouse's. This is a sure sign that the major goal of the public information program is being realized: that is, to raise the consciousness of the participants with regard to their hearing problems. The program has served as an advocate for better hearing and optimal use of residual hearing. In a very real sense, these programs could be viewed as prevention because they are designed to accelerate the identification of hearing impairment and to thereby minimize the number of inappropriate decisions resulting from lack of information regarding hearing impairment.

Finally, it is important to establish that audiologists are the most appropriate professionals to conduct these public information programs. Audiology has always assumed the role of public advocate for better hearing. The academic and clinical training of audiologists encompasses a solid grounding in hearing impairment and hearing handicap, as well as in the management of associated communication problems. Their expertise extends to amplification and parent and individual counseling and equips them to guide the hearing-impaired person through the rehabilitative process. Table 5-1 outlines the components of a public information and audiometric screening program.

○ EVALUATION

Based on a management model of *evaluate-plan-implement-reevaluate,* the most crucial stage of the rehabilitative process is *evaluation.* The major functions of an evaluation in this context are: (1) to assess the handicapping effects of the hearing impairment, especially in terms of communication; and (2) to gauge the success of the rehabilitative process in terms of the alleviation or reduction of these handicapping effects. This involves a thorough evaluation of both *hearing impairment* and *hearing handicap.*

Assessing hearing impairment requires close cooperation with the medical profession. Audiologic testing involving threshold, suprathreshold, and special procedures is initially conducted to assist the otolaryngologist in diagnosing and treating the possible hearing impairment. In this capacity, the audiologist has served as a referral source for the hearing-impaired person and has provided the physician with a reliable and valid description of the person's response to auditory signals presented in a controlled environment using standard test procedures. When the hearing impairment is nonmedically reversible and a communication problem exists, the evaluation of hearing handicap is initiated through further testing and through the reinterpretation of previously administered tests.

Chapters Three and Four contain a detailed discussion of possible evaluation procedures which lend themselves to assessing the effect of a given hearing impairment on a person's everyday life situations. The importance of evaluation at this stage of the rehabilitation process is to generate a comprehensive description of problem areas in order to plan a tailor-made

TABLE 5-1
Components of a Public Information and
Audiometric Screening Program

1. Early identification
2. Medical referral
3. Community lectures and programs
4. Radio and television presentations
5. Prevention of sustaining and increasing hearing handicap

TABLE 5-2
Components of the
Evaluation Process

1. Hearing impairment
2. Medical referral
3. Communication effects
   (a) Receptive
   (b) Expressive
   (c) Response to auditory failure
4. Vocational
5. Family impact

management program. Table 5-2 outlines the essential components of an effective evaluation process.

An evaluation procedure such as that described in Table 5-2 is not seen as an integral part of the standard battery of tests administered to all hearing-impaired persons. The additional testing is only appropriate when audiologic involvement extends beyond the identification and description of the hearing impairment. These persons comprise a small percentage of the audiologist's adult case load, but clearly they will need a management program to help them develop effective communication. This constitutes the remediation process and includes amplification considerations as well as (for some people) communication strategy sessions.

○ DEVELOPING A PLAN

The evaluation process will have generated a profile of hearing impairment and handicap. It will have identified a number of potential communication difficulties experienced by the hearing-impaired person. These difficulties are generally associated with (1) the intensity of the message; (2) speech discrimination; (3) the environment, including background noise and the communication situation; and (4) response to auditory failure. In order for a management program to be relevant and to sustain interest, it must initially be centered around the hearing-impaired person's perceived problem areas. As the program progresses, insights regarding the validity of these perceptions will emerge and activities can be modified to better reflect the true picture of the handicap.

One approach to planning a rehabilitative program of initial relevancy is to begin by discussing with the hearing-impaired person the results of the audiometric and self-report procedures in terms of communication breakdowns. This allows the hearing-impaired person to begin gaining some insight into his or her situation and provides the clinician with the opportunity to introduce the proposed management program in terms of the person's specific hearing problems. It also provides the person with the

opportunity to indicate which problems are of sufficient importance to be
included early in the rehabilitation program.

More importantly, the initial interview can provide an excellent opportunity to begin judging the validity of the clinician's and client's impressions
of the overall handicap. What persons say about their responses on the
self-report scales and how they react to the communication situations identified and to their overall communication performance in those settings will
help the clinician to begin the long process of sifting out the true from the
perceived management needs of the client.

The rehabilitative process has begun with the initial interview. If this
interview is conducted systematically and in a caring manner, it can have
great therapeutic value. It can set the stage for an optimistic and cooperative
period of working toward improved communication. Above all, the interview categorizes the impairment in terms of specific communication problems and what can be done about them.

At this point a specific management program is outlined, and hopefully
the hearing-impaired person agrees to participate. It is important to establish that only a small portion of the audiologist's case load will require an
extensive management program. For many, it will be sufficient to pursue
amplification with appropriate hearing aid orientation, using the evaluation
procedures to assess the success of hearing aid adjustment. In addition, the
discussion regarding the handicapping effect of the hearing impairment will
serve to identify problem areas and their solutions. For example, most
clients report that having the HPI reviewed with them is quite enlightening.
They are amazed to learn what they are or are not doing to control their
listening environment. Some begin changing their communication behavior
on their own. One woman decided on the spot to discontinue playing the
hi-fi in her home as background music when she hosted bridge parties to
see if that would improve her ability to follow the conversation.

A smaller group of people will continue to experience difficulty adjusting
to their hearing aids and/or will experience considerable difficulty in various
communication situations. They will require additional rehabilitative services. For this group, attending an aural rehabilitation group can be beneficial.

## ○ AURAL REHABILITATION GROUPS

The general purpose of aural rehabilitation groups is to provide
supportive and substantive help to persons having communication problems associated with their hearing impairments. The focus is on communication breakdowns, where and with whom they typically occur, and what can
be done about them. The goal is to analyze auditory failures and to develop
concrete behaviors which result in improved communication.

The *group discussion* format is preferred. It provides a dynamic setting in which the interaction between peers (hearing-impaired persons), family members, and the group leader (the audiologist) generates productive discussions and, most importantly, solutions to communication problems. The group serves to affirm the hearing-impaired person's general situation (he or she is not alone) and, through the varied comments made by the group members, highlights the numerous ways in which the same communication situations have been handled. Properly structured, the group emerges as a source for many solutions and a setting for introducing new topics and discussing communication situations specific to that particular group. In many ways, each group emerges with its own unique character, raising similar discussions but handling them in its own unique manner. Barker, Cegala, Kibler, and Wahlers (1979) suggest that an important characteristic of small groups (of three to fifteen persons) is their potential for sharing information. Figures 5–1 and 5–2, reproduced from their book *Groups in Process: An Introduction to Small Group Communication* (pp. 6 and 7), illustrate the potential exchange of original ideas between a dyad (two-person group) and a three-person group. They write:

> [Perhaps the most] . . . important distinction is in the potential for information sharing and exchange. Figures [5–1 and 5–2] illustrate differences in the number of original combinations of ideas possible between a dyad and a three-person group. The different shadings represent areas in which new combinations of ideas are possible by putting members together with original ideas and allowing them to interact.
>
> What this means in real-life discussion groups is that if member A has an idea which is not fully developed, it is possible that member B might be able to provide some insight on the basis of previous training or experience. However, by adding the background and experience of both member B and member C, we increase the possibilities of adding valuable information *four* times. As group members are added, the potential for new combinations of ideas among members increases geometrically (i.e., increases several times the actual number of members added). Of course, there is a point of diminishing returns (probably at about fifteen participants) in which adding other members is of little (or negative) value, because possibilities for interaction are limited. It is at this point that the group ceases to have a basic quality of the *small* group: potential for interaction with every member of the group. (pp. 6–7)

Dyad (One Combination)

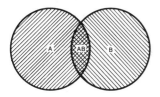

FIGURE 5–1 Dyad—One Combination. (L. Barker et al., *Groups in Process: An Introduction to Small Group Communication.* Englewood Cliffs, N.J.: Prentice-Hall, Inc., 1979, p. 6. Reprinted by permission.)

Basic Small Group
(Three-Person, Four Combinations)

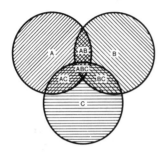

FIGURE 5–2 Basic Small Group—Three-Person, Four Combinations. (From Barker et al., p. 7. Reprinted by permission.)

In addition to increasing their potential for information exchange, a group of people who share a common concern (i.e., hearing handicap) can provide each other with considerable mutual support and comfort. As the group discussions progress, it becomes increasingly apparent that there are more similarities than differences between the communication problems associated with hearing impairment. This discovery has a reassuring effect and considerable therapeutic overflow. Webster (1977), in discussing the value of working with a group of parents of hearing-impaired children, writes:

> A more important rationale for the decision to see several parents in one group is based on . . . the fact that there are similarities among all parents: Those whose children have handicaps share many of the same concerns, aspirations, ideas, and emotions as all other parents. If it is the business of counseling to help parents to deal with these aspects of their lives, as this writer believes it must be, then it can be quite beneficial to group one parent with others. Through interaction with other parents, each may feel less alone, realizing that others cope with similar problems and share similar feelings of frustration or success. Furthermore, parents learn a great deal from each other, sometimes more than they learn from counselors. Opportunity for parental learning is another reason that many counselors want to offer opportunities for multiperson interaction. (p. 64)

Close, cohesive groups of the type being described in this chapter also provide the group members with an opportunity to make direct social comparisons in an attempt to validate their communication behavior. Festinger's (1954) *social comparison theory* contends that when people are not able to validate their own opinions, abilities, and performance by objective, nonsocial means, they compare them with those of others around them. The group can provide an excellent situation in which to make direct social comparisons of appropriate and inappropriate communication behaviors.

In conclusion, the group discussion format, coupled with lectures and communication activities, is considered the most economical, efficient, and effective approach to helping the adult with an acquired hearing impairment. For an in-depth discussion of the numerous rewards of the group process, the reader is referred to Michael Argyle's *The Psychology of Interpersonal Behavior* (1978).

### group leader

The ultimate success of the group lies with the audiologist serving as the group leader. It is the responsibility of the leader to create an atmosphere conducive to free and easily flowing discussion. The audiologist must facilitate discussion by bringing out those persons who are reluctant to talk and at the same time inhibiting the one or two people who might tend to dominate the discussion. The group leader must be a good listener, must convey respect for all participants as capable and creative thinkers, and must establish the belief that many of the important discussion topics will come from the group and not from the audiologist. The audiologist will serve as a discussion facilitator and resource person whose expertise is in the area of hearing impairment and hearing handicap and who has insights gained through experience with other aural rehabilitation groups. The joint participation of the group members and the audiologist should ensure that the issues discussed will be pertinent and that the solutions offered will be practically and theoretically sound.

An accepting group environment such as this is often conducive to introducing a variety of topics which are not always tied to hearing impairment and associated communication problems. It will be important to establish early that the discussion is to be centered around communication and that when it strays, it will be the leader's responsibility to guide the discussion back to the group's main concern.

A word of caution is in order. There is a danger that readers will assume that they must be specialists in the group process: that is, accomplished group facilitators or counselors. That is not the intention of this writer. While a working familiarity with counseling theory and practice will serve the clinician well, it is not a prerequisite to conducting successful aural rehabilitation groups. As stated earlier, the groups' goals and activities are communication-centered, and the audiologists' training in their own discipline will serve them well. Clinicians are encouraged to follow their basic professional inclinations in developing procedures to facilitate discussion and to promote change in communication behavior. Many of the procedures used in regular clinical settings will lend themselves quite well to larger group settings. For those readers who wish to pursue more information about the group discussion process as it is used in the field of communication disorders, Elizabeth J. Webster's *Counseling with Parents of Handicapped Children* (1977) is strongly recommended. Webster's creative interweaving

of counseling theory, group discussion process, and parental communication behavior has direct application to conducting aural rehabilitation
groups. Her point of view is reflected throughout this chapter.

### session structure

While the content and activities will vary from session to session,
each meeting should have the same format so that the participants can
predict the structure from one session to another. From the standpoint of
verbal communication hearing-impaired persons function considerably better in such structured situations. Being able to anticipate the activity (e.g.,
topic under discussion, open discussion, coffee break, etc.) is one of the
most effective ways to fill in the information gaps created by faulty hearing.
The standardized structure of the sessions will provide an ongoing vehicle
to demonstrate this important point to the group participants. As they begin
to appreciate the structure and come to realize how it facilitates their success
in following what is being said, they may begin to incorporate a similar
structure into their own daily communication settings. For example, a par-
ticipant may call the host or hostess of a dinner party to ask the names of
the other guests. Being able to anticipate the names of the guests will put
less strain on the person's hearing during the initial introductions. This
communication strategy is developing a *preparatory set,* and it is strongly
recommended for hearing-impaired persons.

The general format suggested for each session might be as follows:

1. Discussion of homework assignment.
2. Formal presentation of previously announced topic.
3. Open discussion of issues raised in the formal presentation.
4. Social break.
5. Communication strategy activity.
6. Assigning of homework and discussion of the next session's activities.

This group structure represents a blend of several ingredients found in
most traditional instructional approaches. These ingredients include (1) the
presentation of content (through lectures, films, etc.); (2) supervised group
discussion; and (3) activities (role playing, etc.) which highlight issues made
in the lectures or which introduce new content areas.

The group typically meets once a week for six to eight weeks, depending
on the size of the group. Each session is approximately two hours long. Most
people will attend only one set of sessions; the rare person may choose to
attend a second set. Beyond this point, clinical experience suggests that

further assistance is best provided through individual contacts. Those needing further help are often persons who have acquired severe bilateral hearing impairments and/or who are having considerable difficulty accepting their new hearing status. Referral for psychological consultation in conjunction with individual aural rehabilitation sessions is often a productive management route to take.

### group members

The total number of members comprising the group will vary with demand and with the group leader's individual preference. The larger the group, the less opportunity for all members to participate in the discussion portion of the group's activities. An ideal group is about fourteen in number, with no fewer than six and no more than sixteen.

Each hearing-impaired person should be urged to bring a family member or close friend. This person should be someone who is in close contact with the hearing-impaired person and who talks with him or her often. This is an important ingredient in the whole rehabilitative process. Hardick (1977) requires that a normally hearing person accompany the hearing-impaired person. As we know, even with optimal use of amplification and excellent communication strategies, hearing-impaired persons will not be transformed into normally hearing persons. They will continue to have communication failures as a result of their hearing impairments. They will always need the compassionate understanding and support of the people in their immediate environment. Hardick (1977) writes, "The worst enemy the hearing-impaired person has are those well-intentioned, advice-giving, normal-hearing family and friends." Family members and friends often give advice without any real understanding of what it means to have a hearing impairment. This can be minimized by including the family member or close friend in the discussion of the hearing impairment and its handicapping effects from the beginning. This person should learn what can and cannot be done to improve the communication skills of the hearing-impaired person. The role of each person in the rehabilitative process gradually emerges. Through this combined effort, the chances are greater for some real changes to occur.

An added reason for including family members or close friends is to provide the group with a normally hearing person's perspective. Over time, there will be numerous comparisons made between auditory failures experienced by the hearing-impaired members and those experienced by the normally hearing members. The similarities and differences between the kinds of auditory failures and the ways they are handled will become evident. What will emerge is that both groups experience auditory failures and that both groups can learn from each other as to how they can be handled. However, it will also become quite evident that the frequency of these auditory failures is much higher for the hearing-impaired persons and that this alone carries significant consequences.

These exchanges create an environment in which hearing-impaired persons have an opportunity to discuss their communication problems with the normally hearing persons who play significant roles in their lives. This mutual understanding of hearing handicap has far-reaching positive ramifications.

There are no well-established criteria for selecting persons to make up a particular group. Hardick (1977) prefers matching the group members on the basis of amount and duration of hearing loss, age, and socioeconomic level. Another approach is to organize the group according to communication problems as reported by one or more of the evaluation procedures discussed in Chapter Four. By using performance as the major parameter, one can group together persons who perceive that they have similar communication problems. This would produce the most homogeneous groups.

The above criteria must only be viewed as preferred criteria and not as prerequisites to the formation of successful aural rehabilitation groups. Those who conduct these groups must confront the real-world situation of having to form groups on the basis of who is available. Considerable success can be achieved with fairly heterogeneous groups.

On the other hand, there are certain persons who acquired hearing impairments as adults who do not fit well into any group. For example, those persons who acquired sudden severe bilateral hearing losses are best worked with initially on an individual basis. They may eventually be included in a group setting if they progress to a point where such a multi-speaker situation would be more reinforcing than frustrating. Another category consists of adults with unilateral hearing impairments. This population has specific communication difficulties (Giolas and Wark 1967) which are best handled on an individual basis.

### group activities

As stated earlier, the long-term goal of aural rehabilitation is to help the hearing-impaired adult realize optimal communication. The group structure strives to accomplish this by providing the hearing-impaired person with a variety of information and experiences. These include (1) information about hearing, hearing impairment, and its handicapping effects; (2) practice with new compensatory communication strategies; and (3) discussion with hearing-impaired and normally hearing persons with regard to their thoughts about hearing impairment. The basic theme running through all the sessions is that of *self-help.* The overall goal is to help the group members become aware of the many things they themselves can do to improve their communication effectiveness. They are encouraged to analyze communication breakdowns in terms of (1) that portion which is primarily the result of the hearing impairment, (2) that portion which is mostly the result of poor listening habits, and (3) that portion which is primarily the result of an adverse listening environment. The solutions will be a natural outcome of this analysis.

An example of a condition which is primarily the result of the hearing impairment is when the disorder renders a speech signal both less intense and less clear. A logical solution, in part, to these problems is appropriate amplification.

An example of a condition which is mostly the result of poor listening habits is when the hearing-impaired person is not paying attention or is not willing to ask for something to be repeated in hopes that the general meaning will emerge as the conversation progresses. Prior to acquiring the hearing impairment the person could use these strategies quite successfully because of the physiologic, acoustic, linguistic, and situational cues provided by normal hearing. However, these cues are now considerably reduced, and careful listening habits must be developed to compensate for their loss.

An example of an adverse listening environment is one in which there is fairly loud background music (e.g., a restaurant). A competing signal of this sort often has a deleterious effect on speech intelligibility. The easiest solution to this problem is to ask that the music be turned down or to plan ahead and choose a quieter restaurant in which to meet. Hearing-impaired persons report that many establishments are willing to cooperate when they understand the reason.

The members of an aural rehabilitation group should repeatedly be shown the value of having a *plan* when approaching any communication situation. It should be emphasized that they can no longer count on their hearing to overcome the adverse listening environments they may encounter. An example of such a plan was introduced earlier in the case of the hearing-impaired person who called to learn the names of the other guests attending a dinner party. These plans will vary with each situation and can be quite elaborate or as simple as informing another person of one's hearing impairment. These plans will be discussed further in the section dealing with developing compensatory communication strategies.

Finally, all group activities should be designed to make hearing-impaired persons active listeners, persons who have experienced success in many communicative situations by manipulating the environment to their own advantage. While the activities will vary from group to group in terms of specific content and emphasis, several basic areas will most likely be covered at one time or another. Each of these areas is designed to provide the group members with information and group support to experiment with a variety of plans in order to deal with common communicative situations in their daily lives. These areas are (1) optimal use of auditory cues, including hearing aid orientation, and (2) communication strategies, including use of visual cues, manipulation of the environment, and response to auditory failure.

### optimal use of auditory cues

For persons with normal hearing, the auditory modality has played the primary role in most of their mental development. Through the spoken message, complicated information has been transmitted to facilitate the acquisition of language, speech, academic, and vocational skills. The ease with which this takes place is due in large part to the multiple cues provided by verbal as well as nonverbal communication processes. These multiple cues are referred to by some as *redundancy cues;* they are redundant in that there are more cues than are needed to comprehend the message (Miller 1951). The message therefore becomes predictable, and it is this predictability which makes this mode of information transmission so powerful.

The primary cues contributing to the predictability of the spoken message are in the form of physiologic, acoustic, and linguistic parameters. Boothroyd (1978) offers the following example to illustrate how all three of these parameters act to assist in the perception of the sentence, *I bought some new shoes.*

1. The listener heard this with two ears. One would have sufficed (physiologic redundancy).

2. He heard the complete acoustic spectrum. A small portion would have sufficed (acoustic redundancy).

3. Clues to the final consonant were to be found in the consonant itself and in the formant transitions and duration of the preceding vowel (phonetic redundancy).

4. [Z] is one of the few phonemes that can be added to [ʃ uː] and still make a meaningful word (lexical redundancy).

5. The word "some" implies that the last word will be a plural (syntactic redundancy).

6. "World knowledge" tells us that shoes come in pairs (semantic redundancy).

This concept is further supported by numerous studies which demonstrate that it takes considerable message degradation before a major portion of the message cannot be predicted. Giolas, Cooker, and Duffy (1970) demonstrated that it was necessary to remove 40% to 50% of the key words from a group of colloquial sentences before subjects were unable to predict the whole sentences. Other studies showed similar results with words and words in sentences (Miller et al. 1951; Rosenzweig and Postman 1958). Ross, Duffy, Cooker, and Sargeant (1973) illustrated the contribution of prosodic features to the identification of emotion. Their subjects were able to identify the correct emotion expressed, even when the message was filtered at 500 Hz low-pass with an 18 dB per octave cutoff. Add to this the contribution of visual and situational cues in context, and the predictability quotient of any given verbal message is enhanced.

It is this phenomenon of speech predictability that assists persons who acquired hearing impairments in adulthood in compensating effectively, even though many auditory cues are diminished as a result of the disorder. With the help of amplification, many of the physiologic and acoustic cues are restored. Add to this an established internal language structure, special attention to situational cues, and a good preparatory set, and the hearing-impaired adult is often able to function satisfactorily in most listening situations. The remediation process is designed to communicate this information to the hearing-impaired person.

Given that the major parameter of a hearing impairment is intensity reduction as a function of frequency, the basic foundation of the remediation process is *amplification*. The more of the speech message that is received, the more content cues become available to the listener. Consequently, appropriate hearing aids emerge as the single most important component of an aural rehabilitation program for this population.

***Hearing Aid Orientation.*** The appropriate use of amplification is so important to a remediation program that the ultimate effectiveness of the program is dependent upon successful hearing aid use. Clinicians know of too many hearing-impaired persons who are not wearing their hearing aids at all or who are using them improperly. This is primarily a function of poor management. A carefully designed program of hearing aid orientation (HAO) must be an integral part of an aural rehabilitation program. The goal of such a program should be to help hearing-impaired persons receive optimal benefit from their personal hearing aids. The HAO program may take many forms, depending upon the client's needs and the particular audiological setting. It may be an integral part of the hearing aid evaluation service. It may be a separate service in the form of a *hearing aid clinic* offered to all persons for whom a hearing aid is recommended. In some instances, HAO may be a part of the program of aural rehabilitation groups such as those under discussion. In any case, the HAO program should include some basic elements so that it will provide an opportunity for the audiologist to handle most of the problems typically encountered by new hearing aid wearers. In other words, a systematic program of HAO must be routine if it is going to meet the comprehensive needs of the hearing-impaired adult.

There are two prerequisites to an effective HAO program. The first is a careful evaluation of the person's candidacy for a hearing aid. This involves a thorough otological and audiological assessment, with a clear statement from the physician that there are no medical contraindications for fitting the person with a hearing aid. The second prerequisite is an appropriate hearing aid evaluation, selection, and fitting. This service will vary from clinic to clinic but should include serious consideration of binaural amplification, earmold acoustics, and a trial period. Whenever possible, the hearing aid evaluation should be conducted with custom-fitted earmolds.

When the hearing aid has been selected, the first two steps of the HAO program are (1) to introduce the mechanics of using that particular hearing aid and (2) to provide a general orientation to the phenomenon of amplification through a hearing aid. These can be done in a variety of ways but must be done early in the person's experience with amplification. It is important that there be ready access (even if by phone) to the audiologist during these early days of adjusting to the hearing aid. Too much is known about what can go wrong during this crucial adjustment period for the audiologist to trust the process to chance or to some assumed natural progression of events. Snags in this adjustment period can include (1) inappropriate mechanical use of the hearing aid (earmold insertion, volume setting, batteries, or telephone switch); (2) inappropriate wearing habits (insufficient use or poorly selected listening situations); and (3) outright psychological resistance to wearing the hearing aid at all. Sometimes resistance to wearing a hearing aid only emerges as persons are confronted with the reality of their situation and find themselves making up excuses as to why they should not wear it (e.g., it doesn't help, it's too noisy, it's too uncomfortable, etc.). Should this occur, it is important that these feelings be dealt with prior to the purchase of the hearing aid.

One of the ways to facilitate adjustment is to provide a systematic plan for assessing the effectiveness of the hearing aid during the trial period. This plan can be as elaborate or as simple as the situation requires, but it must not be random. It can include pretesting and posttesting with one of the self-report procedures discussed in Chapter Three or it can be a simple set of suggestions as to what to look out for while wearing the new hearing aid.

In any case, at least one follow-up visit prior to purchase is essential. Involving a family member in the entire process can promote not only a better adjustment but greater mutual understanding.

HAO is an important stage in the rehabilitation of the hearing-impaired person and it should be treated as seriously and systematically as the earlier stages of audiological assessment and hearing aid evaluation. In any case, prospective hearing aid users should never be sent out with new hearing aids and told to call if they need help. They deserve more.

For those persons who experienced difficulty adjusting or for those whom the audiologist, based on audiological evaluation, anticipates will have special problems, a more elaborate program may be in order. Such persons may be good candidates for aural rehabilitation groups. In this setting, they can be given the opportunity to experiment with several hearing aids during the sessions. They will have the opportunity to observe others functioning successfully with hearing aids and to listen to the successful users' comments regarding their initial and current thoughts about wearing a hearing aid. Many of the subjects covered in the group presentations and discussions may help clear up some fears and misconceptions the resisters have about wearing a hearing aid. Most importantly, they may begin to deal openly with their resistance to wearing a hearing aid. Such an experience may well move such persons in the direction of trying amplification again, or it may convince them that they are not ready. In either case, they have been spared buying a hearing aid that they probably would not wear.

In summary, consideration of amplification is an important step in the aural rehabilitation of persons who have acquired hearing impairments as adults. The information provided by the auditory mechanism, the acoustic and linguistic message, and the visual and situational cues are enhanced dramatically if the acoustic parameters of the message are optimally restored. In most cases, appropriate hearing aid selection, fitting, and minimal orientation will suffice. For a smaller group of people, a more elaborate orientation program may be needed. These persons may benefit from participation in an aural rehabilitation group. A sample HAO program is outlined in Table 5–3.

### communication strategies

Optimal use of residual hearing through the successful use of a hearing aid will not completely eliminate auditory failure. Auditory failure occurs as a result of uncorrectable distortion of the spoken message due to

TABLE 5–3
Sample Hearing Aid Orientation Program

1. Prerequisites
   (a)   Hearing aid candidacy considerations
   (b)   Hearing aid evaluation, including selection and fitting

2. Introduction to the hearing aid
   (a)   How the hearing aid operates (volume switch, batteries, etc.)
   (b)   Amplification through a hearing aid (advantages and limitations)

3. Assessing the effectiveness of the hearing aid (during trial period)
   (a)   Observations of performance with and without the hearing aid
   (b)   Evaluation of the family member or close friend
   (c)   Pre- and postamplification measurements with self-report procedures
   (d)   Follow-up phone calls and clinic visits
   (e)   Joint meeting to make final decision

4. Handling special problems in hearing aid adjustment
   (a)   Frequent follow-up clinic visits during trial period
   (b)   Participation in aural rehabilitation groups

5. Long-term follow-up
   (a)   Telephone call in three months
   (b)   Clinic visit in six months

the organic hearing impairment and due to adverse environmental conditions. It becomes the responsibility of the hearing-impaired person to develop strategies to compensate for such difficulties. These strategies can be grouped into three categories: (1) use of visual and situational cues; (2) manipulation of the physical environment; and (3) constructive response to auditory failure.

These communication strategies are best introduced and developed in a group setting, where discussion and role playing with two-person or three-person subgroups can be used to demonstrate the principles involved. The emphasis placed on each category of strategies will vary and depends upon the group members' needs.

**_Use of Visual Cues._** One of the more productive compensatory communication strategies used in difficult listening situations is increased reliance on the nonverbal cues inherent in all communication settings. This strategy is based on the assumption that lip movements, facial expressions, gestures, and situational cues offer meaningful supplementary information regarding the content of the conversation. Coupled with the amplified auditory cues provided by the hearing aid, the visual cues accompanying oral communication can certainly enhance the process of decoding the auditory message. Consequently, group activities should be developed to help the group members become more aware of nonauditory cues. This heightened awareness is not difficult to develop and becomes more or less natural as its value is experienced.

Several activities similar to the three listed and described below are usually conducted in one of the early auditory rehabilitation group meetings to illustrate the general advantages of using nonverbal cues. Subsequent activities will center on more specific visual cues. Consistent with the goal of educating both the hearing-impaired persons and their families in the rehabilitation process, all group members are invited to participate in these activities at one time or another.

1. Two group members are asked to sit with their backs to each other and carry on a conversation. Then they and the rest of the group discuss their impressions of what happened. The same conversation is repeated with the same pair facing each other in a normal position. The discussion following the repetition of the conversation often highlights the general contribution of visual cues.

2. Two other people are asked to carry on a conversation under two conditions: the first time using minimal visual cues (minimum lip movements, reduced facial expressions, no hand gestures, etc.) and the second time in a more natural manner. The discussion that follows often points out the benefits derived from watching the speaker more closely, especially his or her face.

3. Two additional people are asked to hold a brief conversation. Prior to initiating the conversation, they are each assigned roles (e.g., physician and patient, real estate agent and prospective homebuyer, etc.). The content of the conversation should be consistent with these roles. The discussion that follows often demonstrates how content can be anticipated on the basis of situational cues. There are obviously many variations of this activity.

The value of activities of this type lies in the discussions that follow. Time should be allowed for the participants in the conversations to express their impressions. However, the whole group should also be encouraged to report their observations. The group leader will play an important part in setting the stage during the initial attempts with these activities. However, this involvement will diminish as the group becomes comfortable with this form of role playing.

The three sample activities described above deal with visual and situational cues on a very general level. It is probably appropriate at this point for the group to discuss lipreading per se. As a matter of fact, it will be almost impossible not to. Regardless of how the group's goals were presented, some group members are there for the specific purpose of learning to lip-read. Most likely, all the group members at this point are overestimating the contribution of lipreading to understanding conversational speech and at the same time underestimating the benefits derived from observing other nonverbal cues. These issues must be dealt with head-on and in a number of ways. The group must be helped to put the roles of various nonverbal cues in their proper perspectives. At a fairly elementary level, the advantages and limitations of lipreading should be pointed out, and several examples should be cited or activities conducted to illustrate each of them. While most persons included in this target population will seldom need to depend upon lipreading exclusively, clues obtained from watching the lips are obviously available. Many potential acoustic confusions can be avoided by a combination of contextual and visual cues. The possible confusion between the acoustically similar verbal requests, "Pass the cheese" and "Pass the peas," could be avoided because of the obvious visible differences between *cheese* and *peas.* Contextual cues would not help to differentiate between *cheese* and *peas,* but visual cues would. Helping people become aware of the probability of this type of confusion will go a long way toward motivating them to watch the speaker. On the other hand, the limitations of depending upon lipreading alone are best illustrated by turning down the sound of the television set and suddenly noticing how little can be gleaned from the silent lip movements on the screen. Even with a familiar program which one has been watching and listening to for quite a while, the words and phrases escape one. Hardick (1977) proposes the following outline for a discussion to acquaint the group with the issues surrounding lipreading:

1. Deterrents to complete understanding of speech visually.
   (a) Visual factors and the effects of aging.
   (b) Factors related to the code, i.e., rate, homopheneity, and varying visibility of phonemes.
   (c) Factors related to the speaker.
   (d) Factors related to the environment, i.e., lighting, distance, and distractions.
   (e) Factors related to the lip-reader.
   (f) Factors related to problems of measurement of lipreading alone or in combination with acoustic energy.

2. Positive aspects.
   (a) Almost all people can read lips to some extent.
   (b) Linguistic factors, i.e., predictability of topics, of words within sentences, and of sentences upon previous sentences.
   (c) That it is best done in conjunction with acoustic energy available to the hearing impaired.

Following a discussion of the role that lipreading actually plays in communication, lipreading activities per se can be included as part of the total rehabilitation process. In addition to directing attention to visual and situational cues, these activities provide an excellent opportunity to teach a general approach to communication. For most groups, this latter goal emerges as the primary purpose for including lipreading activities in the group sessions. A description of a simple lipreading activity will illustrate this point.

Six sentences are written on the chalkboard. The sentences share a common theme or topic (e.g., the weather). In order to familiarize the group with how the sentences appear visually, the group leader says each sentence to the group in the order in which it appears on the chalkboard. Special care is taken to ensure that the group is aware of which sentence is being said. Pairs of sentences are identified and one sentence on a pair is said. The group is asked to identify the correct sentence in each of several pairs. As the group experiences success with this task, the number of sentences comprising the response set is increased until it includes all six sentences. Voice should be used throughout this activity. It provides the most natural conditions for using visual cues. Because the goal of this activity is to provide practice in using visual cues or to teach some other communication strategy, background noise or reduced voice volume may be employed to simulate difficult listening conditions.

The real value of an activity of this type does not lie in whether the group members were able to lip-read the message. It lies in providing the group leader with an opportunity to observe how various group members are approaching the communication situation. Do they give up when they have not understood the first few words, or do they keep trying to look for contextual cues? Do they state what they thought was said and ask for confirmation? Do they ask for the whole sentence to be repeated? Do they take a guess? All of these strategies and others are typically displayed in a lipreading activity. They are also responses common to all communication settings. Some are effective, and others are counterproductive and should not be used. The lipreading activity provides a real-life situation in which to demonstrate the preferred communication strategies. With simple modifications of this basic lipreading activity, additional communication strategies of general applicability can be introduced and practiced. Following are guidelines for developing lipreading activities.

### Guidelines for Lipreading Activities

I. *Rationale.* Lipreading activities are conducted with persons who have acquired a hearing impairment in adulthood for the reasons listed below.

    A. Lipreading activities stimulate awareness of visual and situational cues in the communication setting.

    B. They provide practice using visual and situational cues as a supplementary communication strategy.

    C. They provide an activity in which the hearing-impaired person's approach to speaking-listening situations can be observed.

II. *A basic activity.* A group of sentences, phrases, or key words are written on the chalkboard and used as a basis for working on one or all of the above goals. The message is centered around a common theme and the difficulty of the task is varied as a function of the group's proficiency or the specific goals of the activity. Some suggestions for varying the difficulty of the task are listed below.

    A. Begin with single topics (e.g., baseball).

    B. To increase difficulty add more topics (e.g., sports in general).

    C. Start with short, easily recognizable sentences, and increase length gradually.

    D. Begin by giving many cues (reduced response set), and decrease them gradually (increased response set).

    E. Go from sentences to whole stories, varying the number of cues offered.

    F. Provide for early and continued success. It is important that a positive attitude toward the effective use of visual cues be developed. The overall goal is not so much to teach lipreading per se but rather to have the group experience the value of visual cues in general.

III. *Specific goals.*

    A. Develop activities which illustrate the contributions of situational and contextual cues, gestures, facial expressions, etc.

    B. Provide experiences in observing various speakers from different views and distances.

    C. Discuss the importance of good lighting, proper distance, and looking at the speaker.

Erickson (1974) has described a set of strategies that are designed to improve communication. While they are specifically designed to improve speechreading, they develop an approach which can apply to the total communication process. Following is the list:

1. Watch the speaker—not just his lips, but everything he does, expressions, gestures, and so forth.

2. Check the seating arrangement. This is particularly true in group situations. Don't sit where the speaker will have bright lights behind him. The resulting eyestrain will make speechreading hard, and it will also put the speaker's face in a shadow. It is always best to have your back to the light. In small, informal groups, this is also important. If the room is arranged with a sofa faced by two or three chairs, it is better to sit in one of the chairs in order to have a better view of all the other speakers. If you choose the sofa, the persons on both sides of you will be difficult to speechread. In an auditorium or similar situation, sit close enough to see as well as hear as much as possible.

3. Learn the topic being discussed. When we know what a person is talking about, it is easier to follow the conversation. By following the trend of main ideas, one can contribute to the conversation and avoid making guesses that are far from the topic. When entering a group late, always ask, "What's being discussed?"

4. Learn to look for ideas rather than isolated words. This is the hardest thing a speechreader has to do. With hearing, following ideas is natural. We don't pay attention to any specific words, we just seem to hear and synthesize. The speaker stresses the key words to make them stand out to the listener with normal hearing, an aid to following ideas. While the speechreader may not be able to take advantage of every word a speaker says, with many speakers he can become especially aware of changes in rhythm, stress, timing, and gestures that indicate the words being emphasized and the changes in meaning. By keeping alert for key words in the sentence, the speechreader can follow ideas, even if he misses some of the "verbal filling" from adverbs, prepositions, and other descriptive parts of speech. Nouns and verbs are the most important parts of speech. The other parts of speech embellish or add details that are not vitally essential. To prevent confusion, we are not suggesting that people omit various parts of speech when talking to the hard of hearing, but rather that speechreaders will do better if they do not try to identify every word. As skill advances, more details will become apparent.

5. Use the clues from the situation to help get meanings. The idea is often spelled out by the actual situation. One may also anticipate what vocabulary or phrases will probably be used. The speechreader must recognize and make use of all details in the situation.

6. Stay aware of current events. When we know something about a topic we can more readily recognize the key words, names, and so forth. Because people talk about what is on television and in the news, it will be helpful to read the daily newspaper and to be aware of the programs many people may watch, even if you don't watch television.

7. Keep informed of your friends' interests. Most of our friends have favorite topics. Much as we might desire a change, it is actually a blessing because limited content makes speechreading easier.

8. Try to relax. Don't strain to get every word or syllable. It's not important to understand every word as long as you get the idea. In fact, when you try too hard and get too tense, this will interfere with your ability to speechread.

9. Don't be afraid to guess. Some instructors call it "intelligent guessing." If we know the topic and pick out key words, we can automatically guess the rest of the speech. Some persons won't permit themselves to guess. They have to be sure; consequently, they are constantly getting lost. While they are trying to figure out a word or a phrase, the speaker has continued to talk. Meanwhile, the speechreader who is afraid to guess is concentrating on only one word at a time. By the time he has figured out the introductory remarks, the speaker has completed the story.

10. Be flexible and ready to change your mind when necessary. Because some words may look the same, you will need to get the word clues in the rest of the sentence.

11. Remember, you will usually be using your remaining hearing in combination with your speechreading ability. You can get clues from both channels and use them together to understand the speaker. This will vary with each hard-of-hearing person, depending on his hearing loss or how much a hearing aid helps. Also, situations will vary; you may have to rely on speechreading in some situations more than others.

12. Inform your friends that you are studying speechreading. Tell them it will help you if they don't shout or exaggerate their lip movements when they speak. They also might make a special effort not to cover their mouths and to make sure you can see their faces when they are talking.

13. Keep your sense of humor. There are times when you may confuse a word or subject and feel a little foolish. You may have to say "I sure was off on that word!" and then resume the conversation. As speechreading skills increase, this will happen less often.

14. Watch your own speech. If you talk softly, shout at others, or slur your words together, you are not presenting the model of good speech you would like others to use when talking to you.

15. Don't be afraid of speechreading. Let it become a friend. Like all good friendships, let it develop slowly. It is a skill that requires much practice, not just during lessons, but in everyday living.*

In conclusion, lipreading activities provide a fine opportunity to teach communication strategies that are available to the hearing-impaired adult. In addition, they create natural situations in which to practice these strategies under the supervision of the group leader. Little or no attention need

*J. G. Erickson, *Speech Reading: An Aid to Communication* (Danville, Ill.: The Interstate Printers & Publishers, Inc., 1978), pp. xi–xiv. Reprinted by permission.

be paid to whether there is improvement in lipreading per se. What should be attended to is whether group members are improving in their approach (i.e., developing effective communication strategies) to deciphering the auditory-visual code. Consequently, no formal pretests or posttests in lipreading are administered. This would place too much emphasis on lipreading and would be inconsistent with the group's goals of placing lipreading in a broader context. The assessment of visual cues obtained during the evaluation stage of the aural rehabilitation program is used to identify general areas to be stressed in the group sessions.

***Manipulation of the Environment.*** Environmental conditions such as background noise, lighting, number of people talking, and distance from the speaker can contribute to auditory failure. Whenever possible, these conditions should be manipulated to improve communication efficiency. Following are some guidelines which a hearing-impaired person can follow to improve communication settings.

1. Effect a relatively noise-free environment. This includes requesting that background music be turned down or off, closing doors to minimize corridor noise, and requesting meeting rooms with good acoustics.
2. Secure the most advantageous position relative to the speaker(s). It is always wise to arrive early so that you can have the option of sitting close to the chairperson at meetings, up front at lectures, public hearings, church, etc., and in a position to see all speakers.
3. At informal gatherings limit the number of speakers you engage in conversation at one time. One-to-one conversations are easier than group conversations.
4. Correct poor lighting conditions in order to facilitate the use of all nonverbal cues. Dimly lit restaurants are prime examples of poor lighting conditions. There are often tables that are better lighted than others.
5. Encourage the use of public-address systems when they are available.

Manipulation of the environment is part of the overall *plan* recommended for hearing-impaired persons as they enter specific communication situations. Such plans include analyzing the upcoming situation and developing a *preparatory set* regarding what might be said. Following are three examples drawn from this writer's previous experience with clients.

1. Mr. X enjoyed going to the movies. But he found that even though he wore a hearing aid, he could not always count on hearing well because of poor amplification systems, background music, minimal visual cues, etc. Therefore, he made it a habit to read several reviews of the movie prior to attending. These reviews usually provided enough information about the theme and action to increase his chances of guessing correctly when his hearing failed to provide the information.

2. Ms. Y is a member of her town council. As her hearing became worse, she found she was not able to function as well as she once did during the monthly council meetings. She improved her situation by meeting with the mayor for lunch prior to the monthly meeting and discussing the meeting's agenda. By knowing in advance the topics to be discussed, Ms. Y improved her chances of being able to follow what was being said.

3. Mr. Z found that in informal situations it was helpful for him to bring along someone who understood his hearing difficulty and who could help him keep up with the discussion. The *buddy system* can easily be used with a spouse or close friend and is usually quite successful.

*Response to Auditory Failure.* The consequences of an auditory failure often result directly from the person's response to that failure. If something is done to correct the situation, the consequences are mostly negated. An example of this is when a person misses a point being made, asks for it to be repeated, and the conversation continues. A problem only occurs when an auditory failure goes unchecked and subsequent misunderstandings of what was said develop. Therefore, hearing-impaired persons must develop a repertoire of responses to auditory failure. Following, some fairly successful responses are described.

1. When you are aware that you missed something that was said, ask for it to be repeated. Repeat the portion you heard to facilitate the flow of the conversation.

2. If someone is talking unusually softly, adjust the volume of your hearing aid to hear that person better.

3. Whenever possible, inform the speaker that you have a hearing impairment and suggest what he or she can do to help you understand.

4. Avoid pretending you understood what was said. It will only confuse things later.

5. If you cannot interrupt the speaker, ask someone near you to fill you in on what you did not hear.

6. Even though you feel you are missing a lot, keep trying to follow the discussion. Some nonverbal or situational cues will often emerge to get you back on the track.

7. It is helpful to ask someone near you to alert you to changes in the topic of conversation.

### individual sessions

As the group sessions progress, it often becomes desirable to meet with some of the group members individually to discuss issues or communication strategies specific to their individual needs. These sessions often provide an opportunity to isolate nonproductive strategies being used which are not common to the group as a whole and which, therefore, are not being highlighted in the group sessions. Individual sessions are also times when more personal issues associated with hearing impairment may be discussed. While these sessions are not always needed, in some cases they prove to be an important factor in the individual's progress toward becoming a more effective communicator.

The overall goals and principles governing the clinician's behavior in the individual sessions are identical to those established for the group sessions. In both situations the clinician is interested in helping persons with a hearing impairment develop effective compensatory communication strategies. The major difference between the two situations lies in the number of people involved in helping to identify the solutions. Webster (1977) does not find it useful to talk in terms of individual sessions and group sessions. She argues that both situations represent an interaction between two or more people and that the ingredients of this interpersonal interaction are the same regardless of how many people are involved. In this context, Webster defines a group as ranging from the basic dyad (clinician and client) to multiperson groups (clinician and several clients) such as the aural rehabilitation groups described in this chapter. Following Webster's line of thinking, in an individual session discussion continues to be the basic medium for accomplishing the goals, with the discussion now taking place between two people rather than among several. While all of the basic communication strategies covered in the group sessions are applicable to the individual sessions, the activities must be altered to reflect the number of people involved. Furthermore, the activities planned for the individual sessions should attempt to respond to specific problems which the person is unwilling or unable to bring up in the group sessions.

## SUMMARY

A comprehensive aural rehabilitation program for persons who acquired hearing impairments as adults has been presented. It consists of three major components: (1) public information and audiometric screening, (2) evaluation, and (3) remediation. Each component has been discussed in terms of its rationale, and appropriate sample activities have been presented. The basic theme underlying all three components is that of self-help. Hearing-impaired adults are encouraged to assume responsibility for their own communicative efficiency. The rehabilitative process consists of demonstrating the need for active and aggressive listening and offering practice in it.

Table 5–4 represents an outline of the remediation process.

**TABLE 5–4**
The Remediation Process

I.  Developing a plan.
   A.  Evaluation of handicap is essential in planning management.
   B.  The results of the evaluation must be discussed with the hearing-impaired person.
   C.  From this discussion comes joint participation in developing a management program.

II. Aural rehabilitation groups.
   A.  The purpose of these groups is to provide supportive and substantive help to persons having communication problems associated with hearing impairment.
   B.  Groups have a standard format and an audiologist as leader.
   C.  Groups vary in size and composition, but all members play an active role.
   D.  Group activities vary considerably but must include the following: (1) Optimal use of auditory cues, including hearing aid orientation; (2) Communication strategies, that is, (a) Use of visual cues. (b) Manipulation of the environment. (c) Constructive responses to auditory failure; and (3) Involvement of family members and close friends.
   E.  Reevaluation and development of a new plan.

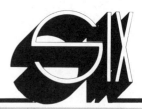

# Aural rehabilitation groups: a sample program

Chapter Five presented a rationale for a comprehensive rehabilitation program. Aural rehabilitation groups were described as an important component for those persons needing follow-up assistance in improving their communication skills. The audiologist was described as playing a central role in developing and conducting these groups. This chapter will present a sample group program. The content and organization of the group sessions described are offered as examples and do not represent a rigid program to be followed with all groups. Developing a management plan for a particular group must be based for the most part on the results of the evaluation process described earlier.

## ○ GROUP MEMBERS AND STRUCTURE

The aural rehabilitation program presented here consists of eight sessions conducted with sixteen members, divided equally between hearing-impaired and normally hearing individuals. Each hearing-impaired person brings along a family member who attends all the sessions. The sessions are held once a week, are two hours in length, and follow the structure outlined in Chapter Five.

The lessons are designed for a group of middle-aged persons, ranging in age from approximately 35 to 65 years. Four members have worn hearing aids for approximately one year and have a number of complaints regarding their hearing aids. Three members are wearing hearing aids for a thirty-day trial period. One member is considering purchasing a hearing aid which was recently recommended by the clinic and has joined the group to learn what others with hearing problems say about amplification.

The audiological evaluations revealed that all group members have sensorineural hearing disorders identified in the last two years. The members' hearing losses range from mild to moderate in degree. The results of the Hearing Performance Inventory (HPI) revealed that the group members reported the following common communication problems:

1. All members reported having some difficulty in understanding speech even when the speaker's voice is loud enough and they can see his or her face. When visual cues are present, their success in these situations ranges from *About half the time* to *Occasionally*. When no visual cues are available, the group's success drops to *Almost never*.

2. Most difficulty was reported with speakers who are females or strangers, in group conversations, and when there is noise in the background. All members identified the group conversation in which people frequently interrupt each other as an extremely difficult listening condition. Other problem situations reported were understanding speech over a public-address system and understanding people who are speaking from another room.

3. Few of the communication strategies assessed in the *Response to Auditory Failure* section of the HPI were employed by the group as a whole. Most noteworthy was the fact that the members seldom (1) adjust their hearing aids, (2) ask for repetition, or (3) inform others of their hearing problems.

4. Six of the members reported that they use more appropriate responses to auditory failures at home than they do at work. All reported similar differences between home and social situations.

5. A number of other conditions are common to several members but not all. These include (1) using fewer communication stragegies with family members, (2) having specific problems at work, and (3) having specific problems in social situations.

## ○ INITIAL INTERVIEW

Prior to beginning the group sessions, an initial interview is held with each group member. The results of the HPI are reviewed in detail with the hearing-impaired person. The main purpose of this session is to jointly identify those communication problems which are of most concern to the individual so that they may be included in the group activities. Furthermore, highlighting the reported problem areas and how they are being handled may motivate some of the potential group members to start making some changes in their behavior on their own and thus may accelerate the management program. Often a family member or close friend is present during this interview. This provides the audiologist with an opportunity to begin validating the responses of the hearing-impaired person.

Following the completion of the initial interview with each group member, an overall plan is developed for the eight weeks. The activities planned for the first week are extremely important. They must address one or more of the concerns reported by *all* the hearing-impaired group members in order to reinforce their initial motivation for enrolling in the group.

## ○ A SAMPLE EIGHT-WEEK AURAL REHABILITATION GROUP PROGRAM

The eight-week program outlined below will follow the session structure described in Chapter Five. The initial session will deviate slightly from this structure in order to introduce the general goals of the program. The basic structure is reproduced here for the reader's convenience.

*General Session Format for Aural Rehabilitation Groups*

1. Discussion of homework assignment.
2. Formal presentation on previously announced topic.
3. Open discussion of issues raised in the formal presentation.
4. Social break.
5. Communication strategy activity.
6. Homework assignment and discussion of the next session's activities.

*First Week*

1.0 *Introduction*
    1.1 Introduction of group members.
    1.2 Setting group goals and ground rules.

2.0 *Formal Presentation*
    2.1 Typical communication problems experienced by most hearing-impaired persons, especially those reported by the group.

        2.1.1 Intensity loss.
        2.1.2 Speech discrimination.
        2.1.3 Communication situations (use examples from self-report data).
        2.1.4 The role of the hearing-impaired person's response to the specific auditory failure.

3.0 *Open Discussion of Formal Presentation*
    3.1 The major objective of this activity in the initial session is to set the stage for an atmosphere conducive to easy conversation between the group members and the leader. The nature of the content is less important at this time.

4.0 *Social Break*
    4.1 The group leader should circulate as much as possible during this initial break and talk with as many of the group members as possible.

5.0 *Communication Strategy Activity*
    5.1 Ask the group to identify difficult listening situations. Write them on the chalkboard and have the group discuss why they are difficult and identify some possible solutions.

6.0 *Homework Assignment*
    6.1 Each group member is asked to identify and describe two situations in which he or she had considerable difficulty during the week. Group members are to chart the situations in terms of:

        6.1.1 With whom they were talking.
        6.1.2 The environmental conditions.
        6.1.3 The purpose of the conversation.
        6.1.4 Why they thought they had difficulty.
        6.1.5 What they did about it.

*Second Week*

1.0 *Discussion of Homework Assignment*
    1.1 Special note must be taken to identify early on those hearing-impaired group members who had difficulty doing the homework

so that they may be responded to individually if the difficulty continues.

2.0 *Formal Presentation*
    2.1 The hearing aid.

        2.1.1 Hearing through a hearing aid.
        2.1.2 The care and operation of a hearing aid.
        2.1.3 Some tips on hearing aid use.

3.0 *Open Discussion of Formal Presentation*
    3.1 This discussion provides the opportunity for many problems and solutions regarding hearing aid use to be raised. Much will be learned from the group members listening and talking to each other. The leader should refrain from providing all the answers.

4.0 *Social Break*
    4.1 This break often provides a good opportunity for group members to ask specific questions concerning problems they are having with their own hearing aids. The group leader should begin noting those persons who may need to be seen for further audiological workup to assess the effectiveness of their hearing aids.

5.0 *Communication Strategy Activity*
    5.1 Two group members are asked to carry on a conversation under adverse listening conditions (e.g., background music). The group is asked to write down how each of the people talking handled the difficult listening situation. A discussion is then held on what was observed.

    5.2 This activity serves as a good introduction to highlight the way responses to auditory failures help or hinder communication.

6.0 *Homework Assignment*
    6.1 Group members are asked to select two listening situations in which they could compare their performance with and without their hearing aids.

*Third Week*

1.0 *Discussion of Homework Assignment*
    1.1 At this point the group leader should be encouraging discussion by those who are not participating very much. If there is someone who is not doing the homework, a nonthreatening personal conversation with him or her (perhaps during the break) is in order.

2.0 *Formal Presentation*
    2.1 The use of nonverbal cues.

        2.1.1 The contribution of lip movements, gestures, facial expressions, and situational cues to the understanding of the verbal message.
        2.1.2 The concept of physiologic, acoustic, and linguistic redundancy (elementary level).
        2.1.3 The benefits and limitations of lipreading.

3.0 *Open Discussion of Formal Presentation*
    3.1 This presentation will stimulate considerable discussion, which will continue to arise in subsequent sessions. The group should be made aware that the use of nonverbal cues will be covered again.

4.0 *Social Break*

    4.1 This is typically the point at which some group members begin to pursue individual conferences with the group leader.

5.0 *Communication Strategy Activity*

    5.1 One or more of the activities described in Chapter Five which are designed to show the advantages of nonverbal cues in general are appropriate at this time.

6.0 *Homework Assignment*

    6.1 Each group member is asked to bring in three to five phrases or sentences common to his or her home or work environment. They will be used in a simple lipreading activity.

*Fourth Week*

1.0 *Discussion of Homework Assignment*

    1.1 This assignment will provide the content with which to introduce a simple lipreading activity. The familiar phrases and sentences will also provide a good lead-in to the use of other communication strategies.

2.0 *Formal Presentation*

    2.1 Communication strategies.

        2.1.1 Manipulation of the environment.

        2.1.2 Constructive response to auditory failure.

    2.2 Many specific suggestions regarding the content of this presentation appear in Chapter Five

3.0 *Open Discussion of Formal Presentation*

    3.1 The group leader may begin directing the discussion toward the group's reported differential use of these strategies in social and work settings.

4.0 *Social Break*

    4.1 If there are some group members who are in their hearing aid trial period or some who are considering getting a hearing aid, this is an appropriate time to check on their progress. They may wish to raise some questions in the group. The break provides a good opportunity to explore this with each of these members personally.

5.0 *Communication Strategy Activity*

    5.1 Using the guidelines for lipreading activities in Chapter Five, a lipreading activity of mild difficulty should be conducted to illustrate one or more of the specific goals outlined in the guidelines.

    5.2 The rationale outlined in the guidelines should be kept in mind throughout these lipreading activities.

    5.3 The hearing-impaired group members should be encouraged to generalize their approach to lipreading to all communication situations.

6.0 *Homework Assignment*

    6.1 Each group member is asked to identify and describe several communication settings in which he or she had little or no difficulty. Group members should document this situation in a manner similar to that prescribed for the first week's assignment. They should pay special attention to the contribution of nonverbal cues.

*Fifth Week*

1.0 *Discussion of Homework Assignment*

    1.1 The purpose of this assignment is to help the group begin identify-
ing strategies that members are using which facilitate communication. The discussion should include as many examples as possible
to illustrate the variety of ingredients comprising a successful communication event. This discussion often becomes a turning point for
many group members as they realize what others are doing to
improve situations similar to those in which they have experienced
difficulty.

2.0 *Formal Presentation*

    2.1 Continuation of fourth week (communication strategies).

    2.2 Stress strategies that have been identified as not being used by the
group.

3.0 *Open Discussion of Formal Presentation*

    3.1 Continuation of the goals established for the fourth week's discus-
sion.

    3.2 It is a good idea for the group leader to review the members'
self-report responses in order to become familiar with their individual profiles. This will facilitate leading the discussion into areas
relevant to all group members.

4.0 *Social Break*

    4.1 The best use of the group leader's time during this break is to check
on the progress being made by those members considering amplification.

5.0 *Communicaton Strategy Activity*

    5.1 Six group members are seated in a circle. Each person is paired
with the person sitting opposite him or her. Each pair is asked
to carry on a conversation, ignoring the other conversations. The
result is three separate conversations going on simultaneously.
The activity is videotaped and analyzed by the group in terms
of how the various participants handled this difficult listening situation. The activity may be repeated with different group members.*

    5.2 This activity presents a graphic picture of which strategies individu-
als are or are not using and is one of the more popular activities.

    5.3 Specific responses to auditory failure that are not being used can
be emphasized.

6.0 *Homework Assignment*

    6.1 By this time all group members should be aware of the necessity
of approaching each communication setting with a plan for improving their ability to understand what is being said. Consequently,
members are asked to identify a communication setting they will
encounter, develop a plan to maximize communication, use the
plan, and analyze its success.

*Courtesy of C. Carman and C. Freedenberg, University of California Hearing and
Speech Center, San Francisco, California.

*Sixth Week*

1.0 *Discussion of Homework Assignment*

    1.1 The discussion of the various plans attempted by the group members will provide the framework for encouraging other plans specific to situations reported by group members. The group leader should use examples of situations common to all members and encourage repetition of this homework activity.

    1.2 The group may wish to devote the remaining homework assignments to this activity. It provides an opportunity for the members to receive help with specific situations especially problematic for them.

2.0 *Formal Presentation*

    2.1 The role of family members and close friends.

        2.1.1 This topic is important because these are the people with whom the hearing-impaired persons spend most of their time and do most of their conversing. Their understanding of the problems of the hearing impaired is vital so that they can contribute to improved communication conditions.

        2.1.2 Review of the options available to the hearing-impaired person.

        2.1.3 Tips on what the family member or close friend can do to facilitate communication.

3.0 *Open Discussion of Formal Presentation*

    3.1 The group leader should be aware that this discussion often produces an increased interaction between the hearing-impaired person and the family member or close friend attending the sessions. This interaction is important and may provide the groundwork for improved handling of communication problems

    3.2 This discussion is also likely to produce comments which stray from the handling of communication situations. The group leader may have to remind the members of the ground rules and goals of the group.

4.0 *Social Break*

    4.1 The break usually becomes an extension of the above discussion.

5.0 *Communication Strategy Activity*

    5.1 Repeat the activity outlined for the fourth week.

    5.2 The activity could be increased in difficulty to challenge the members and provide an opportunity to discuss constructive approaches to various communication situations.

6.0 *Homework Assignment*

    6.1 The hearing-impaired group members should be encouraged to observe what normally hearing persons do when they experience an auditory failure.

    6.2 Those wearing hearing aids on a trial basis should tabulate the situations in which they believe their hearing performance improved as a result of wearing a hearing aid.

*Seventh Week*

1.0 *Discussion of Homework Assignment*

1.1 At this point some attention should be focused on those persons considering amplification.

1.2 The discussion of how normally hearing persons generally handle communication breakdowns lends itself to looking at dissimilarities and likenesses between their experiences with communication breakdown and the experiences of hearing-impaired persons. The conclusion should emerge that the major difference between them lies in the frequency of occurrence.

2.0 *Formal Presentation*

2.1 Hearing and hearing disorders.

2.1.1 Hearing disorders and audiograms.

2.1.2 Hearing handicap.

2.1.3 The role of amplification.

3.0 *Open Discussion of Formal Presentation*

3.1 This discussion can go in a number of directions. It should provide an opportunity for the members to ask all the questions they have about hearing impairment in general and about their own hearing problems in particular.

3.2 In this discussion questions may be raised about the following topics:

3.2.1 The progressive nature of sensorineural hearing impairment.

3.2.2 The hereditary nature of hearing impairment.

3.2.3 The destructive effects of hearing aids on residual hearing.

3.2.4 The value of one versus two hearing aids.

3.2.5 The status of surgery, vitamins, etc., in correcting sensorineural hearing impairment.

4.0 *Social Break*

4.1 This break often becomes an extension of the above discussion.

5.0 *Communication Strategy Activities*

5.1 Group members role-play a number of difficult listening situations and discuss how they could be handled.

5.2 The use of visual, contextual, and situational cues should be stressed.

5.3 Most of the suggested situations should come from the group.

6.0 *Homework Assignment*

6.1 Group members retake the self-report inventory (the HPI) which was taken prior to the first session.

*Eighth Week*

1.0 *Discussion of Homework Assignment*

1.1 This discussion can go in a number of directions. A simple lead-in question such as "How did you feel taking the test this time as opposed to how you felt when you first took it?" will start the discussion.

    1.2 The goal is to help the group members crystallize any insights they believe they have gained from particpating in the group and to discuss how they applied them when retaking the test.

2.0 *Formal Presentation*

    2.1 Summary and review of program goals.

3.0 *Open Discussion of Formal Presentation*

    3.1 The group members may want to use this time to discuss how they benefited from attending the sessions.

4.0 *Social Break*

    4.1 Because this is the last session, the break tends to be longer and more social.

5.0 *Communication Strategy Activity*

    5.1 Review a list of dos and don'ts regarding handling communication situations. A list similar to that developed by Erickson (reproduced in Chapter Five of this book) but modified to reflect an approach to various communication processes is often successful.

    5.2 Discuss and demonstrate appropriate use of a hearing aid.

6.0 *Homework Assignment*

    6.1 Each group member should be encouraged to keep a detailed log of communication situations in which difficulty occurred to be reviewed in the individual follow-up visit approximately a month later.

    6.2 Appointments should be made for the follow-up visit prior to the completion of the session. This is often done by circulating a sign-up sheet with available dates and times.

## SUMMARY

The overall goal of the eight-week program was to provide a setting for hearing-impaired persons to do the following:

1. Obtain systematic information about hearing impairment in general.

2. Identify communication problems specific to their own life situations.

3. Learn how to handle their communication problems through a combination of self-study and information about how other hearing-impaired persons handle similar situations.

4. Share their communication problems and possible solutions with at least one critical person in their lives.

The activities and discussions were designed to highlight the importance of amplification and the use of a variety of communication strategies. The basic concept presented ways that the hearing-impaired person should develop an aggressive approach to all communication situations. The atmosphere of the group sessions should be supportive and accepting and should foster the development of better ways of responding to auditory failure. Whenever appropriate, the formal presentations, activities, and discussions should take into account the group members' reported areas of difficulty.

In conclusion, it is important to emphasize that the program was offered as an example of what might be done from session to session, given a particular group of people. It was not offered as a plan to be followed by all groups. Actually, except for a few issues which probably should be covered with all groups, much of the content of the group's discussions and activities will be influenced by the individuals making up the group, and too much planning in advance is probably not wise.

Finally, this writer believes that there is no better teacher than experience when it comes to leading aural rehabilitation groups. The more groups one conducts, the more adept one seems to become at determining the content and organization of events for a particular group.

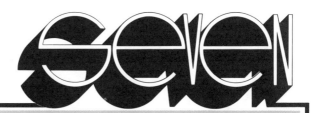

# Special populations

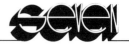

The major concern of this book is the handicapping effect of hearing impairment. The rationale for a comprehensive aural rehabilitation program has been presented. The components comprising the proposed program were discussed in terms of the person who has acquired a hearing impairment as an adult. The sample program outlined in Chapter Six is primarily geared to the adult who can benefit from the group process approach. It is believed that this program will go a long way toward meeting the rehabilitative needs of an underserved segment of the hearing-impaired population. At the same time, there are a number of hearing-impaired adults who present special communication problems which cannot be handled totally within this structure. For them, the evaluation and remediation procedures presented in this book must be modified and/or supplemented in order to be effective. In that these special populations are part of the audiologist's clinical spectrum, a discussion of some of them follows.

## ○ UNILATERAL HEARING IMPAIRMENT

The communication problems experienced by the person with a unilateral hearing impairment are often minimized by the audiologist. Because persons with normal hearing in one ear have functional hearing for the normal acquisition of speech, language, educational, and vocational skills, they are often told that they have normal hearing for all practical purposes. At best, they are cautioned about the possibility that they may have difficulty (1) localizing from which direction sound is coming and (2) understanding speech when the talker is located on the side of the poor ear or when there is background noise present in the listening environment. Beyond this, very little is done to help them maximize their hearing performance in these situations. On the other hand, interviews with unilaterally hearing-impaired persons (Giolas and Wark 1967) revealed that they are extremely aware of their hearing problems and feel they must constantly make special arrangements to ensure optimal listening conditions.

In an attempt to learn more about the specific nature of the problems associated with monaural hearing, Giolas and Wark (1967) interviewed twenty persons with unilateral hearing impairments. The interviews were designed to define the specific situations in which a monaurally hearing person has difficulty communicating. Secondary considerations dealt with the actions taken in response to each situation reported and the feelings associated with these situations. The Critical Incident Technique described by Flanagan (1954) was employed in all interviews.

A total of 100 incidents was reported. These incidents were classified into categories based on similarities in the situations described. Table 7-1 lists the final categories which emerged from the incidents reported, the total number of incidents falling into each category, and the total number of different interviewees contributing incidents to each category.

The eagerness with which persons with unilateral hearing impairments were willing to discuss their hearing difficulties was notable. Ninety percent of the people contacted responded. The feelings associated with various listening situations, as well as general statements made during the course of the interviews, suggested that these individuals experience considerably more communication difficulty than may have been assumed in the past. At

TABLE 7-1
Communication Problem Areas Reported by Persons with a Unilateral Hearing Loss

| Categories | Total Incidents Reported | Number of Persons Contributing to Each Category |
|---|---|---|
| I. Difficulty hearing or understanding speech when it was presented to the impaired ear while the normal ear was partially or fully masked by extraneous noise. | 26 | 16 |
| II. Difficulty hearing or understanding speech when it was presented to the impaired ear while no appreciable extraneous noise masked the normal ear. | 12 | 9 |
| III. Difficulty understanding speech when subject was situated in a setting which contained a great deal of extraneous noise, regardless of whether the stimulus was directed toward the good or the bad ear. | 12 | 9 |
| IV. Difficulty understanding speech when subject was situated in a relatively quiet setting, regardless of whether stimulus was directed toward the good or the bad ear. | 18 | 9 |
| V. Difficulty distinguishing from which direction a given auditory stimulus came in the presence of considerable extraneous noise. | 18 | 11 |
| VI. Difficulty distinguishing from which direction a given auditory stimulus came in a relatively quiet setting. | 12 | 8 |
| VII. Miscellaneous. | 2 | 2 |

Giolas and Wark, 1967.

the conclusion of most of the interviews, the individuals thanked the interviewer for allowing them to talk about their hearing problems. In many cases they pointed out that the interviewer had been the first professional to show an interest in their communication problems.

### problem areas

Extraneous noise was reported as the single most significant factor creating a difficult listening situation. Typical incidents reported were as follows:

> I was at my brother-in-law's house; we had business to discuss. The TV was on and the kids were playing. I couldn't understand a thing he said.
>
> I was at a restaurant for dinner and there was singing and dancing. We sat at a long table with many people around it. I couldn't catch what was being said.

Furthermore, the addition of noise to a given listening situation appears to have its most deleterious effect when it is near or directed toward the good ear. Typical noise sources reported were cars, radios, and air conditioners.

The presence of extraneous noise also appears to interfere with understanding speech regardless of whether it is directed toward the good ear or not. One interviewee put it this way: "There was a room full of people and a lot of noise. I couldn't even understand the person talking right in front of me." Typical situations reported placed the person at a cocktail party, luncheon, or football game.

There is also evidence that not only is localization a problem with monaural hearing but that the problem is compounded by background noise. The greatest number of incidents concerning localization of sound were reported as occurring when the situations were relatively noisy. Typical situations reported were parties, assemblies, and sporting events.

Persons with unilateral hearing impairments also report difficulty in hearing and understanding speech in relatively quiet settings. A typical incident in these categories was:

> I came into the house, which was relatively quiet, and called to a friend, who said, "Yes." I said, "Where are you?" My friend replied, "Right here." I still could not locate her.

A second example was:

> I was sitting on the porch, and a woman drove up and stopped her car 10 to 15 yards away. She asked where my mother was, and I could not understand her.

In this example, distance played an important role. On the whole, distance seemed to be the most common factor creating a difficult listening situation in a relatively quiet setting.

The phenomenon of "head shadow" would appear to be directly related to all three areas of difficulty described above. If, for instance, speech discrimination is as dependent upon relatively high-frequency sounds as is presently assumed, then the form of frequency distortion caused by "head shadow" could have considerable bearing on the understanding of speech.

### actions taken

The uniformity of the actions taken by the interviewees in the various types of listening situations reported was quite noticeable. The actions fell into three general areas. One effective response consisted of altering the immediate environment, such as by moving to a more favorable listening position or eliminating the extraneous noise. A second type of action was to ask the speaker to repeat what had been said. The final and most effective action was for the listener to watch the gestures, face, and lip movements of the speaker. The use of visual cues was reported as being particularly helpful in understanding speech in noisy situations and in localizing speech.

On the basis of these reports, it would seem that a combination of behaviors would greatly facilitate communication in difficult listening situations. This impression is strongly supported by numerous statements made by the interviewees. One such statement was: "I rolled up the window, turned to her, and asked her to repeat it. I watched her face too." However, it was repeatedly reported that it is not always possible to change the immediate environment. Furthermore, if a speaker is not aware of a listener's hearing impairment, the listener often feels obligated to explain his or her hearing difficulty. While this is not considered difficult, most interviewees felt that many situations would be much less threatening if they did not have to worry about explaining their hearing problems to strangers. Many reported that they hesitated to ask strangers to repeat what had been said. Watching the speaker's face and lip movements appeared to be the most effective and convenient action that was taken. Consequently, situations in which the speaker's gestures, face, or lip movements cannot be clearly seen tend to be extremely handicapping. An example of this type of situation is being in an audience and sitting at a considerable distance from the speaker.

### feeling responses

The feelings expressed in response to the various incidents reported were similar in all situations. The majority expressed such negative feelings as embarrassment, annoyance, confusion, and helplessness. It is interesting to note that these negative feelings occur most often in situations where those present are unaware of the individual's hearing impairment.

### clinical implications

It becomes apparent that persons with unilateral hearing impairments need professional assistance. It is evident that persons with monaural hearing do have communication problems and that they tend to have negative feelings about their impairment and the situations in which they experience communication difficulty. One good ear does not afford normal hearing for all practical purposes.

While these persons do not require the extensive aural rehabilitation suggested for the bilaterally hearing-impaired adult, clinical procedures geared to meet the specific needs of persons with monaural hearing must be incorporated into routine clinical programs. Assuming the hearing impairment is medically irreversible, the goals for such procedures should be twofold: (1) the reduction of negative emotions related to the hearing impairment and (2) the development of more effective actions in response to adverse listening situations.

The use of amplification with persons having unilateral hearing impairments has already been suggested by Harford and Barry (1965) and Harford and Dodds (1966). In instances where amplification is appropriate, hearing aid orientation will also be needed as an integral part of the clinical program.

In conclusion, persons with unilateral hearing impairments are at a particular disadvantage in many social communication situations and they do not feel they have normal hearing for all practical purposes.

Special evaluation and remediation procedures which are centered around the specific problems experienced by persons with monaural hearing are needed. At the present time formal procedures are not available and the clinician must improvise. Self-report instruments such as the HPI and the aural rehabilitation groups described in this book are clearly more elaborate than needed for this population; however, they can serve as models for more appropriate procedures.

## ○ SUDDEN HEARING IMPAIRMENT

Generally, the problems associated with a sudden severe bilateral hearing impairment are similar to the problems exhibited by a person with a gradual hearing impairment. However, they are complicated by the sudden, rather than gradual, onset and by the severity of the loss. The initial psychological impact of such a loss is so great that the potential for resistance to nonmedical remediation is marked.

### adjustment pattern

One way to characterize this impact is to discuss it in terms of Ramsdell's primitive, signal or warning, and symbolic levels of hearing (Davis and Silverman 1978). These levels were described in Chapter Two and in part were discussed in terms of persons with sudden hearing impairment. The reader is urged to review this discussion.

In cases of severe bilateral hearing impairment, all three levels of hearing may be affected. The primitive level serves to connect persons with the world around them through hearing. It helps make the environment more alive and multidimensional. When this level is affected, the person begins to experience a general feeling of emptiness and separation from the environment. The world begins to take on an aura of deadness. This feeling is complicated by the simultaneous interference with the signal-warning and symbolic levels. These are more conscious levels of hearing than the primitive level. The signal-warning level provides information about what is going on in the auditory world around us and prepares us to react appropriately. The symbolic level allows us to organize auditory events into meaningful language units for verbal communication. The reduction of hearing at these latter two levels creates feelings of helplessness and cuts a person off from his or her normal mode of speech reception. The net result is a depressed and confused person. One man who experienced rapidly diminishing bilateral hearing put it this way: "Those first few months were awful. I was depressed. I was a mess. The doctor advised me to quit my job and look for one which involved less talking." Given the man's state of mind at the time, this would seem to have been appropriate advice. Fortunately, he was also referred for audiologic help. With early and continued aural rehabilitation, this man is now functioning quite well, is still in the same job, and returns to the audiology clinic annually for follow-up testing and discussion.

The rehabilitative pattern varies from person to person. It is influenced by a number of factors. Some of these factors include: (1) the extent and type of the hearing impairment; (2) the degree to which the person is visually oriented; (3) the person's work situation; (4) the person's general life-style and basic approach to personal problems; and (5) the family's understanding of the problem and overall support.

### remediation

The goals and basic theme underlying aural rehabilitation which were described earlier are directly applicable to persons comprising this population. They must eventually be helped to assume responsibility for their own communication efficiency by becoming active and aggressive listeners. However, it is at the stage of implementation that the remediation program differs.

Initially, considerable time is spent talking with the hearing-impaired person and his or her family. All persons involved are provided with the opportunity to ask as many questions as they wish regarding the status of the individual's hearing, the cause of the impairment, the management plan, and the prognosis for improvement. Throughout this discussion the audiologist strives to play a supportive role. Remedial activities are initiated as soon as possible to provide the person and his or her family with a sense of success and progress. At the same time, the plan should be sufficiently flexible to allow for digression when hearing-impaired persons wish to pursue questions about why they feel as they do, what the future holds for them, and other concerns they may have regarding their hearing. Throughout this management program, the audiologist should always be on the lookout for signs pointing to a psychiatric referral.

It is my experience that persons having acquired sudden hearing impairments are best worked with initially on an individual basis. They are not emotionally or communicatively ready to handle the group setting. Furthermore, their hearing problems are often so much worse than those of any of the other group members that the group experience can be very discouraging when they contrast themselves with others in the group. They may eventually be included in a group setting if they progress to a point where such a multispeaker situation is more reinforcing than frustrating. The one exception to this one-to-one approach is the participation of the family. It is important to hold a group discussion with the family regarding communication problems resulting from a sudden hearing impairment. Furthermore, at least one family member or close friend should be included in most management sessions.

The evaluation procedures described in Chapters Three and Four may be used with this population if their administration and use are modified to meet the adjustment status of the persons being treated. The evaluation procedure should be spread out over time so as to allow remediation to be initiated earlier than is needed with other types of impairments. When some success has been experienced and when a hearing aid is being considered, evaluation procedures such as those discussed in previous chapters may be of value. Owens and Fujikawa (1980) demonstrated the value of using the HPI with severely hearing-impaired adults.

Amplification should always be tried as soon as possible. Its success will depend on a variety of factors including (1) the severity of the loss, (2) its etiology, and (3) the person's willingness to give the hearing aid a fair trial. The trial period should be accompanied by intensive hearing aid orientation activities similar to those described in Chapter Five. The hearing-impaired person must be helped to understand that even though the hearing aid does not restore speech to its preimpairment clarity, coupled with visual and situational cues it can help improve communication efficiency. For some people, it will contribute more to reestablishing the primitive and signal-warning levels of hearing than the symbolic level. One woman with a sudden severe bilateral hearing loss explained her attachment to her hearing aid as follows:

> I know it [the hearing aid] doesn't bring speech in any better, but have you ever vacuumed and not heard the vacuum cleaner noise? It's an eerie feeling! The hearing aid brings in a lot of noises like that and I miss them if I don't hear them.

The activities designed to foster increased use of visual cues that were described in Chapters Five and Six can be productive with this population. Vision symbolizes a significant safety factor and represents a constructive approach to compensating for the hearing impairment. Most importantly, it provides a vehicle through which to present communication strategies applicable to all hearing-impaired persons.

### speech conservation

Speech production is primarily learned and monitored through the sense of hearing. Deterioration of the main factors influencing the intelligibility of speech can occur with a significant hearing impairment. These factors are articulation, voice, and rhythm. Silverman and Calvert (1978) write:

> Defects of articulation usually appear first. Distortion or omission is typical of speech sounds characterized by low intensity and high frequencies, such as /s/, /ʃ/, tʃ/, /f/, and θ. Consonants in the final position in words are particularly vulnerable to erosion. Abnormalities of voice quality, control of volume, and irregularities of speech rhythm may follow as hearing deteriorates. (p. 394)

While speech degeneration is never sudden or total, there may be a gradual erosion of speech intelligibility associated with severe hearing losses. It is possible to minimize this effect. The procedures used will vary depending upon the severity of the loss and the degree to which amplification provides acoustic monitoring cues. The person with a mild to moderate loss will require little extra help beyond good hearing aid orientation to ensure the wearing of a hearing aid. Hearing resumes the role of monitoring channel. On the other hand, a person with a severe to profound loss must develop additional monitoring skills to supplement or replace the poorly functioning auditory mechanism.

A program of speech conservation for persons who have acquired substantial hearing losses postlingually involves three major areas of concentration. These areas are articulation, voice, and emphasis. Silverman and Calvert (1978) state that the main purpose of such a program is to conserve the good speech habits developed prior to the acquisition of the hearing impairment. They suggest that this is accomplished by teaching effective use of kinesthetic cues. Silverman and Calvert suggest that "if training can be started early enough after the hearing loss occurs, no deterioration in speech need result."

The program develops a general understanding of the overall speech production process: i.e., how speech sounds are made from the standpoint of focal articulation points; how the volume and quality of the voice can be modified; and how speech emphasis, in the form of rhythm and melody, can be controlled. A practical approach should be taken to demonstrating all these phenomena. The hearing-impaired person should be helped to experience these changes through systematic practice.

In terms of articulation, the hearing-impaired person is made aware of the kinesthetic distinctiveness of the phonetic elements comprising everyday conversational speech. The clinician identifies those speech messages which have great potential for deterioration and devises activities to provide practice in learning the kinesthetic cues associated with their correct production.

Controlling the volume of the voice is an important part of this program. Because persons with severe sensorineural hearing impairments have lost the normal auditory cues for controlling voice volume, they must develop compensatory skills. These skills involve becoming aware of the bodily sensations associated with proper control of voice volume. This is not an easy task. Silverman and Calvert (1978) suggest two methods for accomplishing this goal.

> The person must first master the ability to talk at each of four or five general levels of loudness. He must learn to shift at will from one level to another. These levels, which are under kinesthetic control, must range from soft speech to very loud speech. Second, the person must study and classify typical sound environments. With the help of his instructor, he can learn what level of background noise he is most likely to encounter in each type of situation. He can then meet the requirements of loudness with reasonable success by speaking at the level (of the five he has learned) that is ordinarily demanded by the situation at hand. Furthermore, an alert talker will notice when his listeners are having difficulty responding to his speech and will raise his voice to the next level. He thus avoids relying rigidly on a set of rules in situations in which it happens that the rules do not apply. (p. 395)

Fine-tuning the rhythm, quality, and emphasis of the spoken message is the third goal of the speech conservation program. This, of course, is a more abstract concept to teach and becomes an ongoing theme throughout the program. The hearing-impaired person must be made cognizant of the need to remain constantly aware of the tendency to speak without inflection. Mechanical methods must be developed to compensate for the fact that hearing does not provide this information. This awareness will provide the motivation for mechanically introducing more life and naturalness into conversational speech.

In summary, a program for persons with sudden hearing impairments provides an opportunity for the individual and his or her family to explore their reactions and questions concerning the disorder. The audiologist plays a supportive role and presents a realistic view of the situation. The benefits and limitations of rehabilitative measures are explained to all concerned. The use of amplification is carefully and cautiously explored. There is no way to predict the length, direction, and nature of this program. It will depend to a great extent upon the motivation of the hearing-impaired person and the support of the family.

## ○ AGE-RELATED HEARING IMPAIRMENT

It is estimated that by the year 2030 approximately 50 million people will be 65 years of age or older. One of the common results of the aging process is a gradual loss of hearing, which is referred to as *presbycusis.* Consistent with the point of view of this book, *presbycusis* is defined as "the handicapping effect of hearing impairment associated with the aging process." *Hearing handicap* was defined in Chapter One as "how the hearing impairment has affected the person's everyday life situation." Presbycusis is therefore seen as a combination of (1) the many physical parameters (including altered hearing) associated with the aging process and (2) the psychological, environmental, and behavioral manifestations of this process. With proper audiological services, the handicapping effects of this hearing impairment can be reduced. Without this assistance, the communication problems associated with presbycusis have an especially detrimental effect on the person's perception of the world.

The aural rehabilitation program outlined in Chapter Five contains three major components: (1) public information and audiometric screening, (2) evaluation, and (3) remediation. The goals associated with these components apply to the elderly as well as to other persons with hearing impairments. In many cases older persons are in a position to avail themselves of the standard audiological service delivery system and do so quite readily and successfully. On the other hand, there are circumstances common to many elderly persons which require adapting current service delivery models to meet the needs of this special population. Prior to presenting these program adaptations, it is necessary to discuss some of the characteristics of presbycusis. Those characteristics which contribute to the understanding of the handicapping effect of this type of hearing impairment and which in turn facilitate audiological rehabilitation will be covered. For an overview of the structural and psychoacoustic parameters of presbycusis, the reader is referred to Willeford (1971).

One of the more obvious clinical characteristics of presbycusis is a reduction in sensitivity to pure tones. Figures 7-1 and 7-2 plot the median hearing losses for men and women, respectively (Glorig, Wheeler, Quiggle, Grings, and Summerfield 1957). This data was obtained as part of the 1954 Wisconsin State Fair Survey. It is apparent that there is a steady loss of sensitivity to pure tones, especially in the higher frequencies, as a function of age. This conclusion has been substantiated with surprising consistency over the years by a number of investigators. The effect of reduced sensitivity on auditory discrimination will be discussed in a later section.

There is also some evidence that persons with hearing difficulty as a function of age can demonstrate a conductive component (Glorig and Davis 1961). Furthermore, this component, reflected audiometrically as an air bone gap, appears at the affected higher frequencies. While there is some controversy over the validity of this phenomenon (Sataloff, Vassalo, and Menduke 1957), it does make sense that the general deterioration associated with the aging process would affect all physical structures of the peripheral auditory mechanism. It follows, then, that presbycusis can have

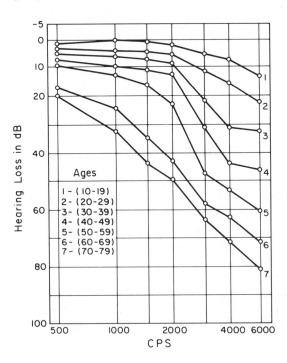

FIGURE 7–1 Median hearing losses of men in the total sample of the Wisconsin State Fair Survey. Data are referenced to ASA, 1951, audiometric zero, left ear only (A. Glorig et al., "1954 Wisconsin State Fair Hearing Survey," Monograph, American Academy of Opthamology and Otolaryngology, 1957. Reprinted by permission.)

both a conductive and a sensorineural component. The obvious rehabilitative value of a nonmedically reversible conductive component in terms of hearing aid use is evident to the experienced audiologist. At the same time, while it may be true that a hearing impairment associated with age can be mixed in nature, it should also be said that there is overwhelming evidence that the hearing impairment will be *primarily* sensorineural.

Schuknecht's (1964, 1974) categorization of four types of presbycusis is an excellent example of the complexity of hearing impairment associated with age. These types are sensory, neural, metabolic, and mechanical. *Sensory presbycusis* is characterized by atrophy of the organ of corti and auditory nerve in the basal end of the cochlea. Schuknecht hypothesized that "the primary locus of degeneration is in the supporting cells of the organ of corti, and the degeneration of the auditory nerve is a secondary phenomenon. The degenerative change is believed to begin in middle age and to progress quite slowly." Hull (1977) writes that this type of presbycusis affects 8000 Hz and above and is the least common of the four types.

*Neural presbycusis* is due to a loss of neurons in the auditory pathways and the cochlea. The effect on hearing usually occurs late in life when the number of functional neurons falls below that required for effective transmission and decoding of neural patterns. It is often characterized by poorer speech discrimination than would be expected according to the measured pure tone thresholds (Goetzinger et al. 1961). Hull (1977) implies that

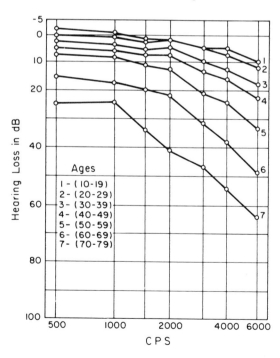

FIGURE 7–2 Median hearing losses for women in the total sample of the Wisconsin State Fair Survey. Data are referenced to ASA, 1951, audiometric zero. (From Glorig et al., 1957. Reproduced by permission.)

adjustment to amplification is more difficult for persons with this type of presbycusis.

*Strial or metabolic presbycusis* is thought to be a result of a defect in the physical and chemical processes by which energy is produced and used by the sense organ (Schuknecht 1964, 1974). Schuknecht (1964) believes that this type of presbycusis is a result of atrophy of the stria vascularis and is genetically determined. The resulting hearing loss is equal for all audiometric thresholds to about 50 dB, at which point speech discrimination becomes affected (Hull 1977). Hull (1977) contends that this type of hearing impairment is often seen where there is a family history with an onset in the third or fourth decade. Hull (1977) also contends that amplification is more noticeably beneficial with persons who have this type of presbycusis.

*Cochlear conductive or mechanical presbycusis* is due to a disorder in the motion mechanics of the cochlear duct, such as changes in the mass and stiffness of the basilar membrane, which produces a progressively descending threshold. General reduced responsiveness of middle ear structures are also considered to contribute to the hearing deficiency associated with this category of presbycusis.

A second very common characteristic of prebycusis is poor speech discrimination. The specific problems comprising this characteristic are similar to those described in Chapter Two with one exception: The problems appear to be inconsistent with the extent of threshold deficit for pure tones, including those of high frequency. In other words, the reduced responsiveness to verbal messages (and probably to nonverbal messages) is more pronounced than what would be expected and typically observed with younger people who have similar audiometric configurations. Hull (1977) describes this phenomenon as consisting of auditory comprehension, cognition, and the sorting of both the phoneme and linguistic features of speech, and he concludes that the cause must be at some level beyond the cochlea and eighth nerve. This phenomenon was first identified by Gaeth (1948), whose description of it still remains one of the more functional ones for clinical purposes. Gaeth named the phenomenon *phonemic regression;* his description is as follows:

1. Otological and audiological findings indicate a hearing loss of the sensorineural type which is either mild or moderate in severity.
2. The threshold shift in hearing for connected speech agrees with the shift for pure tones.
3. There is a greater difficulty in understanding speech, as revealed by appropriate discrimination tests, than the type and severity of loss would lead one to suspect.
4. The patient does not appear to evidence a general decay in mental capabilities paralleling his deterioration in phonemic perception.

5. The patient lacks insight into the quality of his discrimination problem but tends to blame all his troubles on his deficiency in auditory acuity.

6. These symptoms appear more frequently in adults over fifty years of age than in those younger, but a substantial number of the older individuals with hearing losses do not display the difficulty. Therefore, age alone must be ruled out as the causative factor.

Subsequently, Gaeth's observations have been confirmed for the most part by a number of other investigators (Jerger 1973b; Bergman 1976).

### visual perception

As there is a general reduction of responsiveness to auditory stimuli as a function of the aging process, it follows that there may also be reduced responsiveness to visual stimuli. Binnie (1979) writes: "Since all degeneration is found uniformly throughout the brain as a whole, it seems logical to conclude that those control processes which are associated with the visual perception of speech may be less efficient in the geriatric individual (p. 135). A striking example of this is the obvious relationship demonstrated by Shoop and Binnie (1978) to exist between age and the visual comprehension of speech, especially sentences (see Figure 7-3). While the exact cause of this reduced efficiency is not fully understood, the result is often a decreased potential for the optimal use of visual cues in the communication process.

Binnie (1979) has reviewed some of the critical literature on the visual perception of speech. He postulates that

> The causes of visual deterioration among the aged may be related to (1) external changes in the eye, (2) alterations in the condition of the lens, and (3) intraocular conditions. Moreover, problems in visual perceptual performance such as reduced visual memory, retention, and response time may contribute to the overall reduction in visual and auditory-visual speech comprehension.

Binnie also reaches the following conclusions:

1. Visual acuity decreases with age, especially after the age of 50 years (Birren 1964; Weale 1965; Botwinick 1973). The pattern, onset, and rate of change is variable and highly dependent on inherited and environmental factors (Birren 1964; Kalish 1977).

2. Speechreading performance decreases with reduced visual acuity (Lovering and Hardick 1969; Hardick, Oyer, and Irion 1970).

3. Speechreading performance decreases even if acuity is not reduced (Farrimond 1959; Ewertsen and Nielsen 1971; Pelson and Prather 1974; Shoop

and Binner 1978), removing acuity as the primary factor influencing speech-reading ability.

4. Possible explanations offered for the reduced overall visual perceptual performance often seen in some older persons were:

(a) Anatomic changes in the sensory systems may be such as to provide the central nervous system with reduced information from which to make accurate processing decisions.

(b) Central nervous system alterations may interfere with the integration process of information received from one or more senses.

(c) Older persons' responses may be slower, less flexible, resist change from the initial response, and require more exposure time to the stimulus item.

It is important to remind the reader that we have been talking about *group characteristics* associated with persons who have presbycusis. The degree to which *any one* person exhibits *any one* of the problems delineated earlier varies tremendously and is dependent on a host of physical, psychological, and environmental factors. Hull (1977) writes:

Presbycusis, as we currently understand it, then involves: (1) the structural pathology of the aging ear; (2) the auditory processing/comprehension problems seen among aging persons; and (3) the myriad of social/psycho-

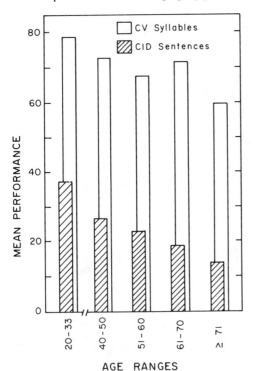

FIGURE 7–3 Histogram comparing distributions of mean performance for CV syllables and CID Sentences among five age treatments. (From Binnie 1979.)

logical problems facing the elderly individual with presbycusis. Schuknecht (1974) has stated that aging is apparently caused by a complex integration of inherited defects; injuries; environmental exposure; accumulation of DNA errors, which results in a reduction of the body's capability of mitosis for repair; the person's genetic makeup; accumulation of pigment; and chemical changes in individual body cells. Schuknecht further feels that presbycusis is precipitated by an accumulation of degenerative changes within the auditory mechanism, but "depending upon heredity, diet, environment, and use."

Unless clinicians remain ever conscious that the aging process is not homogeneous, they will fall into the clinical trap of overgeneralizing and pigeonholing people into stereotypical adjustment patterns. This writer believes that the general handicapping effects of hearing impairment described in Chapter Two and earlier in this chapter are merely potential problems. It is only through careful *evaluation* that we may learn if one or more of these problems are operating in a given individual. While careful and systematic diagnostic procedures are the rule in determining site of lesion in audiology, the same concern for assessing hearing handicap is not generally present. Audiologists must join forces to alter this inconsistency.

Alpiner (1979) builds a strong case for comparing persons with themselves as opposed to comparing groups of persons. He develops a philosophy "of coping with persons on an individual basis regardless of age" (p. 172). He argues that in our attempt to better define the phenomenon of aging so as to develop more meaningful programs, we may have turned the elderly into a "minority group" of sorts, attributing to all group members the same attitudes, behaviors, and potential for change. We must remember that there are clearly people 65 years of age who find growing older a challenge. Life has been good to them and they now find they have more time to pursue their interests, hobbies, and interpersonal relationships with family and friends. Their health and financial status are good. These people must be dealt with as one would an adult of any age.

On the other hand, there are those people who have succumbed to the notion that the world is only for the young. They have health problems and are generally depressed. They live on reduced incomes, have too much time on their hands, many of their friends are deceased, and they do not live where they want to live. Alpiner (1979) contends that if people believe "they are at terminal stages in their lives, if they believe that society has relegated them to have beens, the hearing aids, counseling, and rehabilitative audiology are of no import in everyday living" (p. 170). Aural rehabilitation for these people will, of course, differ greatly from that provided for the first group. The difference is not a function of the age group to which the person belongs, but rather to circumstances specific to that person.

## public information and audiometric screening

The elderly as a group probably know more hearing-impaired people personally than any other group. They most likely have a friend who does not wear the hearing aid he or she has purchased or is constantly complaining about it. Because of a reduction in their overall activity, elderly persons are often not sure whether their hearing is actually getting worse or whether their inconsistent inability to understand is a momentary loss of attention. Their finances are such that they resist incurring new expenses for such things as a hearing evaluation or a hearing aid. They are not sure anything can really be done about their hearing difficulties anyway. What this often means is that the task of convincing elderly persons that they do not have to live with as much of a hearing handicap as they do is difficult. As a result, this makes the public information and audiometric screening programs especially important.

The general format and content of these programs have been discussed in Chapter Five. To a large degree these programs are designed to meet the particular needs of the elderly. A primary key to their success lies in taking them to the people. Holding the lectures, discussions, and screening programs in settings where senior citizens are likely to be present has been quite successful. Many elderly people have transportation problems. It is often difficult for them to afford or arrange transportation to appointments or social events. On the other hand, many have already made arrangements to attend programs and activities such as those offered at a local senior citizen center. In some instances, the center provides transportation on a regular basis. Consequently, integrating a program on hearing can work out quite well. There is no question that there will be better attendance if the program is held in a familiar and often-frequented setting.

Scheduling the time of these programs is also critical. As suggested above, they are best scheduled as part of a regular activity series. People are in the habit of coming at that time, all arrangements are made in advance, and the effort to get to the place is minimal. Scheduling the programs at a separate time, especially at night, is not conducive to a large turnout.

Keeping the cost to the individual to a minimum is also advisable. Whenever possible, the cost should be carried by the center or some other third party. If further audiological services are needed, care should be taken to offer group rates or some other means of reducing the costs.

Up to this point we have been talking about people who are fairly mobile and living independently. There are, of course, many people who are living in health-care facilities of a self-contained nature. Often, these people cannot attend programs outside the facility and in some cases cannot even be transported to the audiology clinic for evaluation. Special procedures and programs must be implemented for these people.

In these situations, in-service training programs for the health-care facility personnel are extremely important. These programs should deal with many of the issues and topics covered by the public information programs and aural rehabilitation groups discussed earlier. The goal is to alert the personnel to the nature of hearing impairment and its associated communication problems. The advantages, limitations, and maintenance of a hearing aid are also reviewed. Finally, ways of communicating with a hearing-impaired person are presented. These programs usually involve all health-care facility personnel. However, it is extremely important to meet separately with those individuals who have frequent contact with hearing-impaired persons to give them specific insight into their patients' hearing difficulties. An outline of an in-service training program is presented below, followed by a list of suggestions which will facilitate communication with hearing-impaired persons.

*Topics Included in an In-Service Presentation on Hearing Impairment for Personnel Working with the Elderly*

1. Incidence.
2. How the ear works.
3. How hearing impairment occurs, with an emphasis on symptoms of presbycusis.
4. Medical treatment.
5. How the elderly person often perceives his or her hearing problem.
6. How the hearing problem appears to the family and friends.
7. Audiological services, including the hearing aid evaluation process.
8. The process of aural rehabilitation.
9. How to communicate with the hearing-impaired person.
10. Other amplification systems for the hearing-impaired person (e.g., telephone and television amplifiers).
11. How to troubleshoot the hearing aid.

*Aids to Communication with Hearing-Impaired Persons* *

1. Be sure your face can be seen easily. Most hearing-impaired persons supplement what they hear with visual cues.
2. The room should be adequately lit and there should be light on your face.
3. Don't try to communicate from behind the person, from another room, or from too great a distance. From three to six feet is the optimal distance for ease in listening.

*Courtesy of Marilyn H. Giolas, M.S. The Southeastern Connecticut Hearing and Speech Center.

4. Speak loudly enough but not too loudly. Shouting often distorts the sound rather than making it clearer.

5. Don't speak too rapidly; to the listener, your words will seem to run together, visually, as well as auditorily. In trying to speak more slowly, be careful not to mouth your words. This destroys the natural look and rhythm of speech, making speechreading very difficult.

6. When you have not been understood, it is wise to rephrase rather than repeat what you've said. Different words or phrases may be more easily understood. In addition, it may be necessary to simplify the message, i.e., shorter sentences, words, etc.

7. For optimal listening, minimize background noise such as television, traffic, or rattling pots and pans. Be willing to turn off the TV, close doors, or even move to another room if necessary.

8. Be sure your listener knows the topic of the conversation and is made aware of a change in topic when it occurs. This aids in speechreading and more intelligent guessing because vocabulary is more predictable.

9. Remember that even though a person wears a hearing aid, normal hearing should not be assumed. It is an important aid, which when combined with the communication strategies listed above, enables the hearing-impaired person to communicate optimally.

### evaluation

As suggested in the introduction to this section, many elderly people can be tested using standard audiological test procedures. This is also true for those procedures used to evaluate hearing handicap which are described in Chapters Five and Six. The evaluation of the handicap phase of an aural rehabilitation program must not be bypassed or short-circuited on the assumption that it is too cumbersome or complicated. This step obviously serves the same function for the elderly as it does for hearing-impaired persons of all ages.

It is recommended that the audiologist begin by assuming that a standard presentation of an evaluation procedure is appropriate and later allow the situation and performance to dictate the modifications. When modifications are necessary, they often result from the need to correct for problems centering around reduced visual perception (e.g., cataracts, central processing); physical problems (e.g., arthritis); and fatigue. In the case of self-report procedures, these modifications often involve presenting the written material in larger print, actually reading the questions out loud, and providing the person with more time to process each item. It may also be necessary to allow more time for the response (Donahue 1971). This is often time-consuming and may involve spreading the test process out over a longer period of time. These modifications are also necessary when reading is a problem, as is the case when English is not the person's primary language. In some instances it may be concluded that a self-report procedure may not be productive. Finally, Alpiner (1978) suggests that persons living in extended-care facilities respond best to self-report procedures presented in an interview format. Zarnoch and Alpiner (1977) developed the Denver Scale of Communication Function for Senior Citizens Living in Retirement Centers to be used accordingly. (See Appendix H for complete copy of this instrument.)

### remediation

The aural rehabilitation groups described in this book are quite appropriate for the elderly person. In many ways, the group process is better suited to this population. The homogeneity of the group's makeup in terms of age, general interests, adjustment patterns, and stage of life often makes this approach more effective than with more heterogeneous groups. Because the aging process in general has often created a general reduction in responsiveness to verbal messages, it is sometimes advisable to reduce the group size. This in turn will reduce the potential number of verbal exchanges and make it easier for the group members to follow the group activities. If the meetings can be held in familiar settings, with members who regularly interact, and at a convenient time, aural rehabilitation groups can be the most rewarding approach to helping the older person with a hearing problem. As with all groups, care should be taken to select activities commensurate with the maturity and experiences of the members. If it is a group of people who have lived in the geographic area for many years, discussions of how things used to be and the history of old landmarks, etc., provide an abundance of materials to implement the communication strategy activities described earlier. In that many elderly people are extremely dependent on family members and/or close friends for social outlets, it is especially important to include family and friends in the group activities. This will facilitate improvement in all aspects of these personal relationships. As indicated earlier, elderly people differ widely in their attitude toward the aging process. The following behavior characteristics described by Mead (1962) and adapted by Alpiner (1979) may help in formulating groups:

1. *Turning to superficial childish satisfactions.* This type of reaction may exist because the older person cannot look ahead to the future. A number of clients attempt to evade focusing on therapy by telling jokes about their childhood. This is not a bad situation, but if the entire focus of the therapy session moves in this direction, it is doubtful that progress in communication function may be achieved. Related to this mechanism is the attitude of clinicians who continually treat adults like children: "Hello, honey, how is the girl today? Don't be sad, you will do better next time." The childish vocal intonations accompanying these types of statements are those we might use with young children in therapy.

2. *Denial mechanism.* Some clients deny old age by resorting to such things as health fads. They may insist that certain vitamins will reverse a hearing loss or make their vision better. They may state that hearing loss is not due to aging but rather to a dietary deficiency caused by not eating the appropriate foods.

3. *Nonacceptance of the aging process.* Some clients do not accept the idea that their disability is caused by aging. Other reasons are sought as causes of the disorder. For example, a person may say that the hearing loss was caused by a serious accident to the head during childhood or that he or she had an illness for which the cause was unknown. The outright refusal to consider the aging process as a possible cause of the problem seems to be the pattern for this particular category.

4. *Inability to cope with the changes of old age.* Some clients see themselves as relegated to a state of depression or apathy. This is not due solely to the hearing loss but is only one traumatic aspect of the multitude of disorders which may accompany aging, such as heart disease and diabetes.

5. *Senility.* The final reaction may result from actual cortical deterioration resulting in senility. This condition precludes the audiologist from engaging in therapy. A caution must be inserted into this category. Some clients who appear to be senile may actually possess severe discrimination problems. They are falsely labeled as senile; Alpiner refers to this particular situation as *pseudosenility.* The situation is often encountered in extended-care facilities in which staffs have not been appropriately trained regarding the manifestations of hearing impairment.

Finally, Binnie (1979) offered the guidelines listed below for working with the elderly in an aural rehabilitation setting. The guidelines are based on his and his colleagues' research in the area of auditory and visual perception of speech as a function of age (Binnie 1974; Binnie 1973; Binnie 1976; Binnie, Jackson, and Montgomery 1976; Shoop and Binnie 1978).

1. Use a standardized film (or videotape) test of speechreading.

2. Check visual acuity of subjects to assure that performance is 20/40 or better.

3. In case history interviews, follow the prevalence of visual difficulties just as one would trace auditory problems, and make appropriate referrals.

4. Administer tests of visual-only performance as well as auditory-visual tests to determine how well the two senses interact.

5. Give ample time for directions and response behavior.

6. Encourage guessing behavior; clients may be closer to the correct response than they think.

7. Inspect results of tests of viseme categorization; these tests may provide a good basis for training in consonant discrimination and recognition.

8. Use sentences and synthetic (environmental) cues which may provide a better estimate of speechreading performance than CV syllables, words, or unrelated sentences.

9. Realize the frustrations of trying to speechread and try to increase clients' motivation.

10. Encourage the use of environmental cues and auditory information to increase overall intelligibility. (p. 173)

**SUMMARY**

The purpose of this chapter was to identify some of the special problems associated with meeting the aural rehabilitation needs of the hearing-impaired adult. No attempt was made to discuss all special populations. This would have been a difficult task and, more importantly, not even desirable. Aural rehabilitation, as presented in this book, is seen as an individualized, tailor-made program. The emphasis on evaluation procedures which stress identifying the specific communication problems experienced by the hearing-impaired person is a good example of this individualized orientation. Further evidence of the individualized approach can be seen in the emphasis on the group process as a rehabilitative method. Hearing-impaired persons are encouraged to assume responsibility for their own communication efficiency through peer interaction. It is in this manner that they will successfully minimize the handicapping effects of their personal hearing impairments.

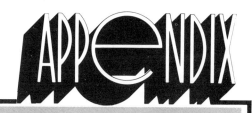

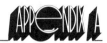

○ GUIDE FOR THE EVALUATION OF HEARING HANDICAP*†

THE GUIDE for the Evaluation of Hearing Handicap has required periodic revisions as new information has become available. The last revision was in 1965. This communication represents a change in the previous formula and details the reasons for the modifications. This is the effort of the American Academy of Otolaryngology Committee on Hearing and Equilibrium and the American Council of Otolaryngology Committee on the Medical Aspects of Noise and represents approximately two years of work. Both committees unanimously endorse the new formula, and the Committee on Hearing and Equilibrium, particularly its Subcommittee on Conservation of Hearing, was responsible for writing and revising the text. The Board of Directors of both the American Academy of Otolaryngology and the American Council of Otolaryngology have approved this modified formula.

### impairment, handicap, and disability

It is important for all physicians to be aware of their role in the evaulation of permanent impairment, handicap, and disability under any private or public program for the disabled. It is equally important for them to have the necessary information to assist them in fulfilling their particular responsibility—the evaluation of permanent impairment and handicap.

In various statements approved by the Committee on Hearing and Equilibrium and its predecessor, the Committee on Conservation of Hearing of the American Academy of Ophthalmology and Otolaryngology (AAOO), the terms "hearing impairment," "hearing handicap," and "hearing disability" have all been employed, often with the intention of conveying substantially the same meaning. However, some confusion has existed because of connotations attached to each of the terms. In this section the definitions are restated to coincide with those approved by the AAOO in 1965.[1]

*American Academy of Otolaryngology Committee on Hearing and Equilibrium, and the American Council of Otolaryngology Committee on the Medical Aspects of Noise, "Guide for the Evaluation of Hearing Handicap," *Journal of the American Medical Association,* 241(1979), pp. 2055–2059. Reprinted by permission.

†Footnote numbers refer to References for the Guide for the Evaluation of Hearing Handicap. References appear on p. 151–152.

**Permanent Impairment.—** A change for the worse in either structure or function, outside the range of normal, is permanent impairment. The term is used here in a medical rather than a legal sense. Permanent impairment is due to any anatomic or functional abnormality that produces hearing loss. This loss should be evaluated after maximum rehabilitation has been achieved and when the impairment is nonprogressive at the time of evaluation. The determination of impairment is basic to the evaluation of permanent handicap and disability.

**Permanent Handicap.—** The disadvantage imposed by an impairment sufficient to affect a person's efficiency in the activities of daily living is permanent handicap. Handicap implies a material impairment.

TABLE A–1
Monaural Hearing Impairment*

| DSHL[†] | % | DSHL[†] | % | DSHL[†] | % |
|---|---|---|---|---|---|
| 100 | 0.0 | 195 | 35.6 | 290 | 71.2 |
| 105 | 1.9 | 200 | 37.5 | 295 | 73.1 |
| 110 | 3.8 | 205 | 39.4 | 300 | 75.0 |
| 115 | 5.6 | 210 | 41.2 | 305 | 76.9 |
| 120 | 7.5 | 215 | 43.1 | 310 | 78.8 |
| 125 | 9.4 | 220 | 45.0 | 315 | 80.6 |
| 130 | 11.2 | 225 | 46.9 | 320 | 82.5 |
| 135 | 13.1 | 230 | 48.9 | 325 | 84.4 |
| 140 | 15.0 | 235 | 50.6 | 330 | 86.2 |
| 145 | 16.9 | 240 | 52.5 | 335 | 88.1 |
| 150 | 18.8 | 245 | 54.4 | 340 | 90.0 |
| 155 | 20.6 | 250 | 56.2 | 345 | 90.9 |
| 160 | 22.5 | 255 | 58.1 | 350 | 93.8 |
| 165 | 24.4 | 260 | 60.0 | 355 | 95.6 |
| 170 | 26.2 | 265 | 61.9 | 360 | 97.5 |
| 175 | 28.1 | 270 | 63.8 | 365 | 99.4 |
| 180 | 30.0 | 275 | 65.6 | 370 | 100.0 |
| 185 | 31.9 | 280 | 67.5 | (or greater) | |
| 190 | 33.8 | 285 | 69.3 | | |

*1. From the audiogram of numerical record of the audiometric test, find the decibel sum the hearing threshold levels (DSHL) of 500, 1,000, 2,000, and 3,000 Hz. Example:

    500   20
  1,000   25
  2,000   35
  3,000   40
  Total     120 DSHL

2. Under the DSHL heading, 120 DSHL (column 1, line 5) equals 7.5%.

3. Computation of percent of hearing handicap: If the monaural percent figure is the same for both ears, that figure expresses the percent hearing handicap. If the percent monaural hearing impairments are not the same, apply the formula:

$$\frac{(5 \times \% \text{ [better ear]}) + (1 \times \% \text{ [poorer ear]})}{6} = \% \text{ hearing handicap}$$

Audiometers are calibrated to ANSI 1969 standard reference levels.

[†] Decibel sum of hearing threshold levels at 500, 1,000, 2,000, and 3,000 Hz.

***Permanent Disability.—*** An actual or presumed inability to remain employed at full wages is a permanent disability. A person is permanently disabled or under permanent disability when the actual or presumed ability to engage in gainful activity is reduced because of handicap and when no appreciable improvement can be expected.

The aforementioned definition of handicap is essentially identical with the definition of "impairment" appearing in the American Medical Association's *Guides to the Evaluation of Permanent Impairment,*[2] namely, "a medical condition that affects one's personal efficiency in the activities of daily living." Disability remains defined as an actual or presumed reduction in ability to remain employed at full wages, and it involves nonmedical factors such as age, sex, education, and economic and social environment. A permanent impairment that is a handicap is, therefore, a contributing factor to, but

## TABLE A-2   Computation of Hearing Handicap

| ANSI 1969 | 100 | 105 | 110 | 115 | 120 | 125 | 130 | 135 | 140 | 145 | 150 | 155 | 160 | 165 | 170 | 175 | 180 | 185 | 190 | 195 | 200 | 205 | 210 | 215 | 220 |
|---|---|---|---|---|---|---|---|---|---|---|---|---|---|---|---|---|---|---|---|---|---|---|---|---|---|
| 100 | 0 | | | | | | | | | | | | | | | | | | | | | | | | |
| 105 | .3 | 1.9 | | | | | | | | | | | | | | | | | | | | | | | |
| 110 | .6 | 2.2 | 3.8 | | | | | | | | | | | | | | | | | | | | | | |
| 115 | .9 | 2.5 | 4.1 | 5.6 | | | | | | | | | | | | | | | | | | | | | |
| 120 | 1.3 | 2.8 | 4.4 | 5.9 | 7.5 | | | | | | | | | | | | | | | | | | | | |
| 125 | 1.6 | 3.1 | 4.7 | 6.3 | 7.8 | 9.4 | | | | | | | | | | | | | | | | | | | |
| 130 | 1.9 | 3.4 | 5 | 6.6 | 8.1 | 9.7 | 11.3 | | | | | | | | | | | | | | | | | | |
| 135 | 2.2 | 3.8 | 5.3 | 6.9 | 8.4 | 10 | 11.6 | 13.1 | | | | | | | | | | | | | | | | | |
| 140 | 2.5 | 4.1 | 5.6 | 7.2 | 8.8 | 10.3 | 11.9 | 13.4 | 15 | | | | | | | | | | | | | | | | |
| 145 | 2.8 | 4.4 | 5.9 | 7.5 | 9.1 | 10.6 | 12.2 | 13.8 | 15.3 | 16.9 | | | | | | | | | | | | | | | |
| 150 | 3.1 | 4.7 | 6.3 | 7.8 | 9.4 | 10.9 | 12.5 | 14.1 | 15.6 | 17.2 | 18.8 | | | | | | | | | | | | | | |
| 155 | 3.4 | 5 | 6.6 | 8.1 | 9.7 | 11.3 | 12.8 | 14.4 | 15.9 | 17.5 | 19.1 | 20.6 | | | | | | | | | | | | | |
| 160 | 3.8 | 5.3 | 6.9 | 8.4 | 10 | 11.6 | 13.1 | 14.7 | 16.3 | 17.8 | 19.4 | 20.9 | 22.5 | | | | | | | | | | | | |
| 165 | 4.1 | 5.6 | 7.2 | 8.8 | 10.3 | 11.9 | 13.4 | 15 | 16.6 | 18.1 | 19.7 | 21.3 | 22.8 | 24.4 | | | | | | | | | | | |
| 170 | 4.4 | 5.9 | 7.5 | 9.1 | 10.6 | 12.2 | 13.8 | 15.3 | 16.9 | 18.4 | 20 | 21.6 | 23.1 | 24.7 | 26.3 | | | | | | | | | | |
| 175 | 4.7 | 6.3 | 7.8 | 9.4 | 10.9 | 12.5 | 14.1 | 15.6 | 17.2 | 18.8 | 20.3 | 21.9 | 23.4 | 25 | 26.6 | 28.1 | | | | | | | | | |
| 180 | 5 | 6.6 | 8.1 | 9.7 | 11.3 | 12.8 | 14.4 | 15.9 | 17.5 | 19.1 | 20.6 | 22.2 | 23.8 | 25.3 | 26.9 | 28.4 | 30 | | | | | | | | |
| 185 | 5.3 | 6.9 | 8.4 | 10 | 11.6 | 13.1 | 14.7 | 16.3 | 17.8 | 19.4 | 20.9 | 22.5 | 24.1 | 25.6 | 27.2 | 28.8 | 30.3 | 31.9 | | | | | | | |
| 190 | 5.6 | 7.2 | 8.8 | 10.3 | 11.9 | 13.4 | 15 | 16.6 | 18.1 | 19.7 | 21.3 | 22.8 | 24.4 | 25.9 | 27.5 | 29.1 | 30.6 | 32.2 | 33.8 | | | | | | |
| 195 | 5.9 | 7.5 | 9.1 | 10.6 | 12.2 | 13.8 | 15.3 | 16.9 | 18.4 | 20 | 21.6 | 23.1 | 24.7 | 26.3 | 27.8 | 29.4 | 30.9 | 32.5 | 34.1 | 35.6 | | | | | |
| 200 | 6.3 | 7.8 | 9.4 | 10.9 | 12.5 | 14.1 | 15.6 | 17.2 | 18.8 | 20.3 | 21.9 | 23.4 | 25 | 26.6 | 28.1 | 29.7 | 31.3 | 32.8 | 34.4 | 35.9 | 37.5 | | | | |
| 205 | 6.6 | 8.1 | 9.7 | 11.3 | 12.8 | 14.4 | 15.9 | 17.5 | 19.1 | 20.6 | 22.2 | 23.8 | 25.3 | 26.9 | 28.4 | 30 | 31.6 | 33.1 | 34.7 | 36.3 | 37.8 | 39.4 | | | |
| 210 | 6.9 | 8.4 | 10 | 11.6 | 13.1 | 14.7 | 16.3 | 17.8 | 19.4 | 20.9 | 22.5 | 24.1 | 25.6 | 27.2 | 28.8 | 30.3 | 31.9 | 33.4 | 35 | 36.6 | 38.1 | 39.7 | 41.3 | | |
| 215 | 7.2 | 8.8 | 10.3 | 11.9 | 13.4 | 15 | 16.6 | 18.1 | 19.7 | 21.3 | 22.8 | 24.4 | 25.9 | 27.5 | 29.1 | 30.6 | 32.2 | 33.8 | 35.3 | 36.9 | 38.4 | 40 | 41.6 | 43.1 | |
| 220 | 7.5 | 9.1 | 10.6 | 12.2 | 13.8 | 15.3 | 16.9 | 18.4 | 20 | 21.6 | 23.1 | 24.7 | 26.3 | 27.8 | 29.4 | 30.9 | 32.5 | 34.1 | 35.6 | 37.2 | 38.8 | 40.3 | 41.9 | 43.4 | 45 |
| 225 | 7.8 | 9.4 | 10.9 | 12.5 | 14.1 | 15.6 | 17.2 | 18.8 | 20.3 | 21.9 | 23.4 | 25 | 26.6 | 28.1 | 29.7 | 31.3 | 32.8 | 34.4 | 35.9 | 37.5 | 39.1 | 40.6 | 42.2 | 43.8 | 45.3 |
| 230 | 8.1 | 9.7 | 11.3 | 12.8 | 14.4 | 15.9 | 17.5 | 19.1 | 20.6 | 22.2 | 23.8 | 25.3 | 26.9 | 28.4 | 30 | 31.6 | 33.1 | 34.7 | 36.3 | 37.8 | 39.4 | 40.9 | 42.5 | 44.1 | 45.6 |
| 235 | 8.4 | 10 | 11.6 | 13.1 | 14.7 | 16.3 | 17.8 | 19.4 | 20.9 | 22.5 | 24.1 | 25.6 | 27.2 | 28.8 | 30.3 | 31.9 | 33.4 | 35 | 36.6 | 38.1 | 39.7 | 41.3 | 42.8 | 44.4 | 45.9 |
| 240 | 8.8 | 10.3 | 11.9 | 13.4 | 15 | 16.6 | 18.1 | 19.7 | 21.3 | 22.8 | 24.4 | 25.9 | 27.5 | 29.1 | 30.6 | 32.2 | 33.8 | 35.3 | 36.9 | 38.4 | 40 | 41.6 | 43.1 | 44.7 | 46.3 |
| 245 | 9.1 | 10.6 | 12.2 | 13.8 | 15.3 | 16.9 | 18.4 | 20 | 21.6 | 23.1 | 24.7 | 26.3 | 27.8 | 29.4 | 30.9 | 32.5 | 34.1 | 35.6 | 37.2 | 38.8 | 40.3 | 41.9 | 43.4 | 45 | 46.6 |
| 250 | 9.4 | 10.9 | 12.5 | 14.1 | 15.6 | 17.2 | 18.8 | 20.3 | 21.9 | 23.4 | 25 | 26.6 | 28.1 | 29.7 | 31.3 | 32.8 | 34.4 | 35.9 | 37.5 | 39.1 | 40.6 | 42.2 | 43.8 | 45.3 | 46.9 |
| 255 | 9.7 | 11.3 | 12.8 | 14.4 | 15.9 | 17.5 | 19.1 | 20.6 | 22.2 | 23.8 | 25.3 | 26.9 | 28.4 | 30 | 31.6 | 33.1 | 34.7 | 36.3 | 37.8 | 39.4 | 40.9 | 42.5 | 44.1 | 45.6 | 47.2 |
| 260 | 10 | 11.6 | 13.1 | 14.7 | 16.3 | 17.8 | 19.4 | 20.9 | 22.5 | 24.1 | 25.6 | 27.2 | 28.8 | 30.3 | 31.9 | 33.4 | 35 | 36.6 | 38.1 | 39.7 | 41.3 | 42.8 | 44.4 | 45.9 | 47.5 |
| 265 | 10.3 | 11.9 | 13.4 | 15 | 16.6 | 18.1 | 19.7 | 21.3 | 22.8 | 24.4 | 25.9 | 27.5 | 29.1 | 30.6 | 32.2 | 33.8 | 35.3 | 36.9 | 38.4 | 40 | 41.6 | 43.1 | 44.7 | 46.3 | 47.8 |
| 270 | 10.6 | 12.2 | 13.8 | 15.3 | 16.9 | 18.4 | 20 | 21.6 | 23.1 | 24.7 | 26.3 | 27.8 | 29.4 | 30.9 | 32.5 | 34.1 | 35.6 | 37.2 | 38.8 | 40.3 | 41.9 | 43.4 | 45 | 46.6 | 48.1 |
| 275 | 10.9 | 12.5 | 14.1 | 15.6 | 17.2 | 18.8 | 20.3 | 21.9 | 23.4 | 25 | 26.6 | 28.1 | 29.7 | 31.3 | 32.8 | 34.4 | 35.9 | 37.5 | 39.1 | 40.6 | 42.2 | 43.8 | 45.3 | 46.9 | 48.4 |
| 280 | 11.3 | 12.8 | 14.4 | 15.9 | 17.5 | 19.1 | 20.6 | 22.2 | 23.8 | 25.3 | 26.9 | 28.4 | 30 | 31.6 | 33.1 | 34.7 | 36.3 | 37.8 | 39.4 | 40.9 | 42.5 | 44.1 | 45.6 | 47.2 | 48.8 |
| 285 | 11.6 | 13.1 | 14.7 | 16.3 | 17.8 | 19.4 | 20.9 | 22.5 | 24.1 | 25.6 | 27.2 | 28.8 | 30.3 | 31.9 | 33.4 | 35 | 36.6 | 38.1 | 39.7 | 41.3 | 42.8 | 44.4 | 45.9 | 47.5 | 49.1 |
| 290 | 11.9 | 13.4 | 15 | 16.6 | 18.1 | 19.7 | 21.3 | 22.8 | 24.4 | 25.9 | 27.5 | 29.1 | 30.6 | 32.2 | 33.8 | 35.3 | 36.9 | 38.4 | 40 | 41.6 | 43.1 | 44.7 | 46.3 | 47.8 | 49.4 |
| 295 | 12.2 | 13.8 | 15.3 | 16.9 | 18.4 | 20 | 21.6 | 23.1 | 24.7 | 26.3 | 27.8 | 29.4 | 30.9 | 32.5 | 34.1 | 35.6 | 37.2 | 38.8 | 40.3 | 41.9 | 43.4 | 45 | 46.6 | 48.1 | 49.7 |
| 300 | 12.5 | 14.1 | 15.6 | 17.2 | 18.8 | 20.3 | 21.9 | 23.4 | 25 | 26.6 | 28.1 | 29.7 | 31.3 | 32.8 | 34.4 | 35.9 | 37.5 | 39.1 | 40.6 | 42.2 | 43.8 | 45.3 | 46.9 | 48.4 | 50 |
| 305 | 12.8 | 14.4 | 15.9 | 17.5 | 19.1 | 20.6 | 22.2 | 23.8 | 25.3 | 26.9 | 28.4 | 30 | 31.6 | 33.1 | 34.7 | 36.3 | 37.8 | 39.4 | 40.9 | 42.5 | 44.1 | 45.6 | 47.2 | 48.8 | 50.3 |
| 310 | 13.1 | 14.7 | 16.3 | 17.8 | 19.4 | 20.9 | 22.5 | 24.1 | 25.6 | 27.2 | 28.8 | 30.3 | 31.9 | 33.4 | 35 | 36.6 | 38.1 | 39.7 | 41.3 | 42.8 | 44.4 | 45.9 | 47.5 | 49.1 | 50.6 |
| 315 | 13.4 | 15 | 16.6 | 18.1 | 19.7 | 21.3 | 22.8 | 24.4 | 25.9 | 27.5 | 29.1 | 30.6 | 32.2 | 33.8 | 35.3 | 36.9 | 38.4 | 40 | 41.6 | 43.1 | 44.7 | 46.3 | 47.8 | 49.4 | 50.9 |
| 320 | 13.8 | 15.3 | 16.9 | 18.4 | 20 | 21.6 | 23.1 | 24.7 | 26.3 | 27.8 | 29.4 | 30.9 | 32.5 | 34.1 | 35.6 | 37.2 | 38.8 | 40.3 | 41.9 | 43.4 | 45 | 46.6 | 48.1 | 49.7 | 51.3 |
| 325 | 14.1 | 15.6 | 17.2 | 18.8 | 20.3 | 21.9 | 23.4 | 25 | 26.6 | 28.1 | 29.7 | 31.3 | 32.8 | 34.4 | 35.9 | 37.5 | 39.1 | 40.6 | 42.2 | 43.8 | 45.3 | 46.9 | 48.4 | 50 | 51.6 |
| 330 | 14.4 | 15.9 | 17.5 | 19.1 | 20.6 | 22.2 | 23.8 | 25.3 | 26.9 | 28.4 | 30 | 31.6 | 33.1 | 34.7 | 36.3 | 37.8 | 39.4 | 40.9 | 42.5 | 44.1 | 45.6 | 47.2 | 48.8 | 50.3 | 51.9 |
| 335 | 14.7 | 16.3 | 17.8 | 19.4 | 20.9 | 22.5 | 24.1 | 25.6 | 27.2 | 28.8 | 30.3 | 31.9 | 33.4 | 35 | 36.6 | 38.1 | 39.7 | 41.3 | 42.8 | 44.4 | 45.9 | 47.5 | 49.1 | 50.6 | 52.2 |
| 340 | 15 | 16.6 | 18.1 | 19.7 | 21.3 | 22.8 | 24.4 | 25.9 | 27.5 | 29.1 | 30.6 | 32.2 | 33.8 | 35.3 | 36.9 | 38.4 | 40 | 41.6 | 43.1 | 44.7 | 46.3 | 47.8 | 49.4 | 50.9 | 52.5 |
| 345 | 15.3 | 16.9 | 18.4 | 20 | 21.6 | 23.1 | 24.7 | 26.3 | 27.8 | 29.4 | 30.9 | 32.5 | 34.1 | 35.6 | 37.2 | 38.8 | 40.3 | 41.9 | 43.4 | 45 | 46.6 | 48.1 | 49.7 | 51.3 | 52.8 |
| 350 | 15.6 | 17.2 | 18.8 | 20.3 | 21.9 | 23.4 | 25 | 26.6 | 28.1 | 29.7 | 31.3 | 32.8 | 34.4 | 35.9 | 37.5 | 39.1 | 40.6 | 42.2 | 43.8 | 45.3 | 46.9 | 48.4 | 50 | 51.6 | 53.1 |
| 355 | 15.9 | 17.5 | 19.1 | 20.6 | 22.2 | 23.8 | 25.3 | 26.9 | 28.4 | 30 | 31.6 | 33.1 | 34.7 | 36.3 | 37.8 | 39.4 | 40.9 | 42.5 | 44.1 | 45.6 | 47.2 | 48.8 | 50.3 | 51.9 | 53.4 |
| 360 | 16.3 | 17.8 | 19.4 | 20.9 | 22.5 | 24.1 | 25.6 | 27.2 | 28.8 | 30.3 | 31.9 | 33.4 | 35 | 36.6 | 38.1 | 39.7 | 41.3 | 42.8 | 44.4 | 45.9 | 47.5 | 49.1 | 50.6 | 52.2 | 53.8 |
| 365 | 16.6 | 18.1 | 19.7 | 21.3 | 22.8 | 24.4 | 25.9 | 27.5 | 29.1 | 30.6 | 32.2 | 33.8 | 35.3 | 36.9 | 38.4 | 40 | 41.6 | 43.1 | 44.7 | 46.3 | 47.8 | 49.4 | 50.9 | 52.5 | 54.1 |
| 368 | 16.8 | 18.3 | 19.9 | 21.4 | 23 | 24.6 | 26.2 | 27.7 | 29.3 | 30.8 | 32.4 | 33.9 | 35.5 | 37.1 | 38.6 | 40.2 | 41.8 | 43.3 | 44.9 | 46.4 | 48 | 49.6 | 51.1 | 52.7 | 54.3 |
| ANSI 1969 | 100 | 105 | 110 | 115 | 120 | 125 | 130 | 135 | 140 | 145 | 150 | 155 | 160 | 165 | 170 | 175 | 180 | 185 | 190 | 195 | 200 | 205 | 210 | 215 | 220 |

Better Ear (sum 500, 1,000, 2,000, 3,000 Hz)

not necessarily an indication of, the extent of a person's permanent disability under workmen's compensation laws. "Impairment" need not imply appreciable handicap and may be used in a more general sense to denote any deviation from normal. The term "handicap" is so useful in this broad sense that the 1965 guide departed from previous use by employing "handicap" to identify a material impairment sufficient to "affect one's personal efficiency in the activities of daily living."

**Evaluation of Permanent Impairment.—** Evaluation of permanent impairment is an appraisal of the nature and extent of a person's illness or injury as it affects structure or function, and it lies within the scope of medical responsibility preparatory to the assessment of permanent handicap and disability.

## TABLE A-2  (Continued)

*Values are based on the following formula:

$$\frac{5 \times \% \text{ impairment of better ear} + \% \text{ impairment of worse ear}}{6} = \text{hearing handicap}$$

The axes are the sum of hearing levels at 500, 1,000, 2,000, and 3,000 Hz. The sum for the worse ear is read at the side; the sum for the better ear is read at the bottom. At the intersection of the column for the worse ear and the column for the better ear is the hearing handicap.

| | | | | | | | | | | | | | | | | | | | | | | | | | | | | | |
|---|---|---|---|---|---|---|---|---|---|---|---|---|---|---|---|---|---|---|---|---|---|---|---|---|---|---|---|---|---|
| 46.9 | | | | | | | | | | | | | | | | | | | | | | | | | | | | | |
| 47.2 | 48.8 | | | | | | | | | | | | | | | | | | | | | | | | | | | | |
| 47.5 | 49.1 | 50.6 | | | | | | | | | | | | | | | | | | | | | | | | | | | |
| 47.8 | 49.4 | 50.9 | 52.5 | | | | | | | | | | | | | | | | | | | | | | | | | | |
| 48.1 | 49.7 | 51.3 | 52.8 | 54.4 | | | | | | | | | | | | | | | | | | | | | | | | | |
| 48.4 | 50 | 51.6 | 53.1 | 54.7 | 56.3 | | | | | | | | | | | | | | | | | | | | | | | | |
| 48.8 | 50.3 | 51.9 | 53.4 | 55 | 56.6 | 58.1 | | | | | | | | | | | | | | | | | | | | | | | |
| 49.1 | 50.6 | 52.2 | 53.8 | 55.3 | 56.9 | 58.4 | 60 | | | | | | | | | | | | | | | | | | | | | | |
| 49.4 | 50.9 | 52.5 | 54.1 | 55.6 | 57.2 | 58.8 | 60.3 | 61.9 | | | | | | | | | | | | | | | | | | | | | |
| 49.7 | 51.3 | 52.8 | 54.4 | 55.9 | 57.5 | 59.1 | 60.6 | 62.2 | 63.8 | | | | | | | | | | | | | | | | | | | | |
| 50 | 51.6 | 53.1 | 54.7 | 56.3 | 57.8 | 59.4 | 60.9 | 62.5 | 64.1 | 65.6 | | | | | | | | | | | | | | | | | | | |
| 50.3 | 51.9 | 53.4 | 55 | 56.6 | 58.1 | 59.7 | 61.3 | 62.8 | 64.4 | 65.9 | 67.5 | | | | | | | | | | | | | | | | | | |
| 50.6 | 52.2 | 53.8 | 55.3 | 56.9 | 58.4 | 60 | 61.6 | 63.1 | 64.7 | 66.3 | 67.8 | 69.4 | | | | | | | | | | | | | | | | | |
| 50.9 | 52.5 | 54.1 | 55.6 | 57.2 | 58.8 | 60.3 | 61.9 | 63.4 | 65 | 66.6 | 68.1 | 69.7 | 71.3 | | | | | | | | | | | | | | | | |
| 51.3 | 52.8 | 54.4 | 55.9 | 57.5 | 59.1 | 60.6 | 62.2 | 63.8 | 65.3 | 66.9 | 68.4 | 70 | 71.6 | 73.1 | | | | | | | | | | | | | | | |
| 51.6 | 53.1 | 54.7 | 56.3 | 57.8 | 59.4 | 60.9 | 62.5 | 64.1 | 65.6 | 67.2 | 68.8 | 70.3 | 71.9 | 73.4 | 75 | | | | | | | | | | | | | | |
| 51.9 | 53.4 | 55 | 56.6 | 58.1 | 59.7 | 61.3 | 62.8 | 64.4 | 65.9 | 67.5 | 69.1 | 70.6 | 72.2 | 73.8 | 75.3 | 76.9 | | | | | | | | | | | | | |
| 52.2 | 53.8 | 55.3 | 56.9 | 58.4 | 60 | 61.6 | 63.1 | 64.7 | 66.3 | 67.8 | 69.4 | 70.9 | 72.5 | 74.1 | 75.6 | 77.2 | 78.8 | | | | | | | | | | | | |
| 52.5 | 54.1 | 55.6 | 57.2 | 58.8 | 60.3 | 61.9 | 63.4 | 65 | 66.6 | 68.1 | 69.7 | 71.3 | 72.8 | 74.4 | 75.9 | 77.5 | 79.1 | 80.6 | | | | | | | | | | | |
| 52.8 | 54.4 | 55.9 | 57.5 | 59.1 | 60.6 | 62.2 | 63.8 | 65.3 | 66.9 | 68.4 | 70 | 71.6 | 73.1 | 74.7 | 76.3 | 77.8 | 79.4 | 80.9 | 82.5 | | | | | | | | | | |
| 53.1 | 54.7 | 56.3 | 57.8 | 59.4 | 60.9 | 62.5 | 64.1 | 65.6 | 67.2 | 68.8 | 70.3 | 71.9 | 73.4 | 75 | 76.6 | 78.1 | 79.7 | 81.3 | 82.8 | 84.4 | | | | | | | | | |
| 53.4 | 55 | 56.6 | 58.1 | 59.7 | 61.3 | 62.8 | 64.4 | 65.9 | 67.5 | 69.1 | 70.6 | 72.2 | 73.8 | 75.3 | 76.9 | 78.4 | 80 | 81.6 | 83.1 | 84.7 | 86.3 | | | | | | | | |
| 53.8 | 55.3 | 56.9 | 58.4 | 60 | 61.6 | 63.1 | 64.7 | 66.3 | 67.8 | 69.4 | 70.9 | 72.5 | 74.1 | 75.6 | 77.2 | 78.8 | 80.3 | 81.9 | 83.4 | 85 | 86.6 | 88.1 | | | | | | | |
| 54.1 | 55.6 | 57.2 | 58.8 | 60.3 | 61.9 | 63.4 | 65 | 66.6 | 68.1 | 69.7 | 71.3 | 72.8 | 74.4 | 75.9 | 77.5 | 79.1 | 80.6 | 82.2 | 83.8 | 85.3 | 86.9 | 88.4 | 90 | | | | | | |
| 54.4 | 55.9 | 57.5 | 59.1 | 60.6 | 62.2 | 63.8 | 65.3 | 66.9 | 68.4 | 70 | 71.6 | 73.1 | 74.7 | 76.3 | 77.8 | 79.4 | 80.9 | 82.5 | 84.1 | 85.6 | 87.2 | 88.8 | 90.3 | 91.9 | | | | | |
| 54.7 | 56.3 | 57.8 | 59.4 | 60.9 | 62.5 | 64.1 | 65.6 | 67.2 | 68.8 | 70.3 | 71.9 | 73.4 | 75 | 76.6 | 78.1 | 79.7 | 81.3 | 82.8 | 84.4 | 85.9 | 87.5 | 89.1 | 90.6 | 92.2 | 93.8 | | | | |
| 55 | 56.6 | 58.1 | 59.7 | 61.3 | 62.8 | 64.4 | 65.9 | 67.5 | 69.1 | 70.6 | 72.2 | 73.8 | 75.3 | 76.9 | 78.4 | 80 | 81.6 | 83.1 | 84.7 | 86.3 | 87.8 | 89.4 | 90.9 | 92.5 | 94.1 | 95.6 | | | |
| 55.3 | 56.9 | 58.4 | 60 | 61.6 | 63.1 | 64.7 | 66.3 | 67.8 | 69.4 | 70.9 | 72.5 | 74.1 | 75.6 | 77.2 | 78.8 | 80.3 | 81.9 | 83.4 | 85 | 86.6 | 88.1 | 89.7 | 91.3 | 92.8 | 94.4 | 95.9 | 97.5 | | |
| 55.6 | 57.2 | 58.8 | 60.3 | 61.9 | 63.4 | 65 | 66.6 | 68.1 | 69.7 | 71.3 | 72.8 | 74.4 | 75.9 | 77.5 | 79.1 | 80.6 | 82.2 | 83.8 | 85.3 | 86.9 | 88.4 | 90 | 91.6 | 93.1 | 94.7 | 96.3 | 97.8 | 99.4 | |
| 55.8 | 57.4 | 58.9 | 60.5 | 62.1 | 63.6 | 65.2 | 66.8 | 68.3 | 69.9 | 71.4 | 73 | 74.6 | 76.1 | 77.7 | 79.3 | 80.8 | 82.4 | 83.9 | 85.5 | 87.1 | 88.6 | 90.2 | 91.8 | 93.3 | 94.9 | 96.4 | 98 | 99.6 | 100 |
| 225 | 230 | 235 | 240 | 245 | 250 | 255 | 260 | 265 | 270 | 275 | 280 | 285 | 290 | 295 | 300 | 305 | 310 | 315 | 320 | 325 | 330 | 335 | 340 | 345 | 350 | 355 | 360 | 365 | 368 |

***Evaluation of Permanent Handicap.***— Evaluation of permanent handicap is an appraisal of the disadvantage imposed by an impairment on the person's efficiency in the activities of daily living.

***Evaluation of Permanent Disability.***— Evaluation of permanent disability is an administrative responsibility based, in part, on medical information. It is an appraisal of a person's present and probable future ability to engage in gainful activity as it is affected not only by the medical factor (permanent handicap) but also by other factors such as age, sex, education, and economic and social environment. Since many nonmedical factors have proved difficult to measure, permanent handicap often becomes the principal criterion of permanent disability.

Determination of disability is an administrative decision as to the worker's entitlement to compensation that should be based on complete medical evaluation and accurate assessment of function using standards that are uniform nationwide and that apply regardless of the manner in which the handicap was acquired.

### historical background information

Sensorineural hearing impairment cannot be assessed in terms of the loss of sensory cells and neurons; instead, some change in function must be measured. The changes in function that are commonly measured are the threshold sensitivity for pure tones and some index of the ability to hear and understand speech. The determination of threshold sensitivity for pure tones in quiet is a standard procedure. However, methods for assessing the ability to understand speech have not been well standardized because the understanding of speech is affected by such variables as vocabulary, education, intelligence, and nature of speech test material, in addition to hearing ability per se.[3]

In the early days of pure tone audiometry, the degree of hearing loss was expressed in terms of the total range of the audiometer (120 dB). This led to the so-called 0.8 rule, since each decibel represented 0.8% of this range.[4] In a medicolegal context, the 0.8 rule was illogical. Normal hearing sensitivity is not a single value but a range of values around audiometric zero. For example, a hearing level of 10 dB is considered normal but would have been rated as corresponding to an 8% hearing handicap under the 0.8 rule. At the other extreme, persons with hearing thresholds considerably below 120 dB cannot hear or understand everyday speech, and the severity of their hearing loss was underrated.

Subsequent efforts[5,6] to find better methods for the evaluation of hearing loss in medicolegal applications led to complex schemes that differentially weighted hearing levels at various audiometric test frequencies according to their relative importance for the hearing of speech. The resulting AMA method proved to be unsatisfactory in practice because of its complexity and because it was less appropriate for sensorineural than for conductive hearing losses.

Further efforts to define hearing loss were divided into two stages. The first stage[7] was to define handicap in terms of hearing for speech: the ability to identify spoken words or sentences under everyday conditions of normal living. This statement anticipated that during the second stage, standardized tests for the hearing of everyday speech would be developed. Specific quantitative recommendations for the determination of handicap would then be proposed. We still do not have such tests.

Other attempts to define hearing loss included studies relating the hearing of one or more forms of speech to the audiometric threshold for pure tones.[8,10] The relative intelligibility of different speech materials was also investigated.[11,12] The AAOO Committee on Conservation of Hearing (now the Committee on Hearing and Equilibrium) and the AMA Committee on Medical Rating of Physical Impairment reviewed the available information and reached the specific recommendations published in guides for the evaluation of hearing impairment (now handicap).[12,13]

The specific recommendations were built on the principles published earlier.[7] Handicap was rated in terms of the ability to hear everyday speech in quiet. In the absence of a good test for hearing speech in quiet, the thresholds for pure tones were used to predict the threshold of hearing for speech. The simplest method for achieving a reasonably accurate prediction of impairment of hearing for speech was to use the average of the hearing threshold levels at 500, 1,000, and 2,000 Hz.[8–10,12] Prediction did not seem to be improved by the inclusion of other frequencies such as 3,000 or 4,000 Hz. Impairment of hearing was calculated from the number of decibels by which the average hearing threshold level exceeded 15 dB American Standards Association (ASA) 1951.[14] Complete or total hearing impairment was set at 82 dB ASA 1951. This value was approximately correct and had the added advantage that percent of impairment could be calculated simply as 1.5% times the number of decibels by which the average hearing threshold levels exceeded 15 dB ASA 1951.

In June 1971 new levels were adopted by the AMA to reflect the change in audiometric zero American National Standards Institute (ANSI) S3.6-1969.[15] The old threshold for hearing impairment of 15 dB ASA 1951 became 25 dB ANSI 1969, and the level for total impairment of 82 dB ASA 1951 became 92 dB ANSI 1969.

The Committee on Hearing and Equilibrium and its Subcommittee on the Conservation of Hearing have periodically reviewed the accuracy of the 1959 guidelines for the hearing of speech and found them appropriate as long as a quiet environment was considered the proper test background. These guidelines do not necessarily apply to the hearing of speech in noisy environments. Quiet was chosen originally for that purpose because it was easier to agree on its definition than on that of a standard noise environment that would simulate an everyday listening situation. However, when the noise level begins to approach the level of the speech signals, as occurs in many everyday listening situations, the 1959 guidelines no longer provide an accurate measure of handicap.[16-18]

The Committee believes that the basis for the calculation of hearing handicap should be altered to reflect a more realistic degree of the understanding of speech, not only in the quiet but also in the presence of some noise. Although a decrease in hearing sensitivity at 3,000 Hz has little effect on hearing speech in quiet,[8-10] it produces a handicap in the presence of noise[16-18] or when speech is distorted.[19-21]

The Committee believes that the hearing threshold level at 3,000 Hz should be included in the calculation of hearing handicap to provide a more accurate assessment of hearing handicap in a greater variety of everyday listening conditions.

### recommendations

The Committee on Hearing and Equilibrium of the American Academy of Ophthalmology and Otolaryngology recommends that the calculation of hearing handicap for adults be derived from the pure-tone audiogram obtained with an audiometer calibrated to ANSI S3.6-1969 standards (Tables 1 and 2). This computation does not apply to children who have not yet acquired language. Hearing handicap is always based on the functional state of both ears.

1. The average of the hearing threshold levels at 500, 1,000, 2,000, and 3,000 Hz should be calculated for each ear.

2. The percent impairment for each ear should be calculated by multiplying by 1.5% the amount by which the aforementioned average hearing threshold level exceeds 25 dB (low fence) up to a maximum of 100%, which is reached at 92 dB (high fence).

3. The hearing handicap, a binaural assessment, should then be calculated by multiplying the smaller percentage (better ear), by 5, adding this figure to the larger percentage (poorer ear), and dividing the total by 6.

Following are examples of the recommended calculation of hearing handicap:

A. Mild to Marked Bilateral Sensorineural Hearing Loss

|           | 500 Hz | 1,000 Hz | 2,000 Hz | 3,000 Hz |
|-----------|--------|----------|----------|----------|
| Right ear | 15     | 25       | 45       | 55       |
| Left ear  | 30     | 45       | 60       | 85       |

1. Calculation of the average hearing threshold level:
   Right ear:

$$\frac{15+25+45+55}{4} = \frac{140}{4} = 35 \text{ dB}$$

   Left ear:

$$\frac{30+45+60+85}{4} = \frac{220}{4} = 55 \text{ dB}$$

2. Calculation of monaural impairment:
   Right ear:
   35 dB–25 dB = 10 dB; 10 X 1.5% = 15%
   Left ear:
   55 dB–25 dB = 30 dB; 30 X 1.5% = 45%

3. Calculation of hearing handicap:
   Smaller number (better ear)
   15% X 5 = 75
   Larger number (poorer ear)
   45% X 1 = 45
   Total, 120÷6 = 20%

Therefore, a person with the hearing threshold levels shown in this audiogram would have a 20% hearing handicap.

### B. Slight Bilateral Sensorineural Hearing Loss

|           | 500 Hz | 1,000 Hz | 2,000 Hz | 3,000 Hz |
|-----------|--------|----------|----------|----------|
| Right ear | 15     | 15       | 20       | 30       |
| Left ear  | 20     | 20       | 30       | 40       |

1. Average hearing threshold level:
   Right ear:

$$\frac{15+15+20+30}{4} = \frac{80}{4} = 20 \text{ dB}$$

   Left ear:

$$\frac{20+20+30+40}{4} = \frac{110}{4} = 27.5 \text{ dB}$$

2. Monaural impairment:
   Right ear:
   20 dB–25 dB = –5 dB; 0 X 1.5% = 0%
   Left ear:
   27.5 dB–25 dB = 2.5 dB;
   2.5 X 1.5% = 3.75%

3. Hearing handicap:
Smaller number (better ear)
0% X 5 = 0.00
Larger number (poorer ear)
3.75% X 1 = 3.75
Total, 3.75÷6 = 1% (rounded off)

Therefore, the hearing handicap is 1%.

C. Severe to Extreme Bilateral
Sensorineural Hearing Loss

|            | 500 Hz | 1,000 Hz | 2,000 Hz | 3,000 Hz |
|------------|--------|----------|----------|----------|
| Right ear: | 80     | 90       | 100      | 110      |
| Left ear:  | 75     | 80       | 90       | 95       |

1. Average hearing threshold level (use 92 dB maximal value):
Right ear:

$$\frac{80+90+100+110}{4} = \frac{380}{4} = 95 \text{ dB}$$

Left ear:

$$\frac{75+80+90+95}{4} = \frac{310}{4} = 85 \text{ dB}$$

2. Monaural impairment:
Right ear:
92 dB (maximum)–25 dB = 67 dB;
67 X 1.5% = 100%

Left ear:
85 dB–25 dB = 60 dB; 60 X 1.5% = 90%

3. Hearing handicap:
Smaller number (better ear)
90% X 5 = 450
Larger number (poorer ear)
100% X 1 = 100
Total, 550÷6 = 92%

Therefore, the hearing handicap is 92%.

**references**

1. Davis H: Guide for the classification and evaluation of hearing handicap in relation to the International Audiometric Zero. *Trans. Am. Acad. Ophthalmol. Otolaryngol.* 69:740–751, 1965. 2. Guide to the evaluation of permanent impairment: Ear, nose, throat, and related structures, AMA Committee on Medical Rating of Physical Impairment. *JAMA* 177:489–501, 1961. 3. Silverman SR, Hirsh IJ: Problems related to the use of speech in clinical audiometry. *Ann. Otol. Rhinol. Laryngol.* 64:1234–1248,

1955. 4. Fletcher H: *Speech and Hearing.* New York, Van Nostrand Co, 1929. 5. Tentative standard procedure for evaluating the percentage of useful hearing loss in medicolegal cases, Council on Physical Therapy. *JAMA* 119:1108–1109, 1942. 6. Tentative standard procedure for evaluating the percentage loss of hearing in medicolegal cases, Council on Physical Medicine. *JAMA* 133:396–397, 1947. 7. Principles for evaluating hearing loss, Council on Physical Medicine and Rehabilitation, abstracted. *JAMA* 157:1408–1409, 1955. 8. Carhart R: Speech reception in relation to pattern of pure tone loss. *J. Speech Disord.* 11:97–108, 1946. 9. Harris JD, Haines HL, Myers CK: A new formula for using the audiogram to predict speech hearing loss. *Arch. Otolaryngol.* 63:158–176, 1956. 10. Quiggle RR, Glorig A, Delk JH, et al: Predicting hearing loss for speech from pure tone audiograms. *Laryngoscope* 67:1–15, 1957. 11. French NR, Steinberg JC: Factors governing the intelligibility of speech sounds. *J. Acoust. Soc. Am.* 19:90–119, 1947. 12. Hirsh IJ, Reynolds EG, Joseph M: Intelligibility of different speech materials. *J. Acoust. Soc. Am.* 26:530–538, 1954. 13. Guide for the evaluation of hearing impairment: Report of the AAOO Committee on Conservation of Hearing (Subcommittee on Noise in Industry). *Trans. Am. Acad. Ophthalmol. Otolaryngol.* 63:236–238, 1959. 14. *American Standard Specification for Audiometers for General Diagnostic Purposes, Z24.5–1951.* New York, American Standards Association, 1951. 15. *American National Standard Specifications for Audiometers, ANSI S3.6-1969.* New York, American National Standards Institute, Inc, 1970. 16. Kryter KD, Williams C, Green DM: Auditory acuity and the perception of speech. *J. Acoust. Soc. Am.* 34:1217–1223, 1962. 17. Suter AH: The ability of mildly hearing-impaired individuals to discriminate speech in noise, EPA 550/9-78-100, AMRL-TR-78-4. US Environmental Protection Agency, 1978. 18. Aniansson G: Methods for assessing high frequency hearing loss in everyday listening situations. *Acta Otolaryngol* 320(suppl): chapters 3 and 5, 1974. 19. Harris JD: Combinations of distortion in speech. The 25% safety factor by multiple-cueing. *Arch. Otolaryngol.* 72:227–232, 1960. 20. Harris JD, Haines JD, Myers CK: The importance of hearing at 3 kc for understanding speeded speech. *Laryngoscope* 70:131–146, 1960. 21. Harris JD: Pure-tone acuity and the intelligibility of everyday speech. *J. Acoust. Soc. Am.* 37:824–830, 1965.

American Academy of Otolaryngology Committee on Hearing and Equilibrium: *Chairman:* Francis I. Catlin, MD. *Committee Members:* Hugh O. Barber, MD; Derald E. Brackmann, MD; Robert W. Cantrell, MD; Richard R. Gacek, MD; Ralph V. Ganser, MD; George A. Gates, MD; F. Blair Simmons, MD; George H. Williams, MD. *Consultants:* Leo G. Doerfler, PhD; Donald H. Eldredge, MD; Joseph E. Hawkins, Jr., PhD; James F. Jerger, PhD; Ralph F. Nauton, MD; Juergen Tonndorf, MD; W. Dixon Ward, PhD.

American Council of Otolaryngology Committee on the Medical Aspects of Noise: *Chairman:* Robert W. Cantrell, MD. *Committee Members:* Meyer S. Fox, MD; Aram Glorig, MD; Donald J. Joseph, MD; William C. Morgan, Jr., MD; Maurice Schiff. MD; George H. Williams, MD. *Consultant:* Francis I. Catlin, MD.

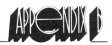

○ A REPORT OF THE AMERICAN SPEECH-LANGUAGE-HEARING
ASSOCIATION TASK FORCE ON THE DEFINITION OF
HEARING HANDICAP*

**introduction**

In 1976, the Executive Board of the American Speech-Language-Hearing Association (ASHA) passed a resolution recommending "that a Task Force on the Definition of Hearing Handicap be appointed to formulate and recommend to the Executive Board a definition of when a hearing impairment becomes a hearing handicap," and this Task Force was formed in early 1978. In recent years, federal and state agencies, government program planners and regulators, third-party payors, and a variety of special interests have looked to the American Speech-Language-Hearing Association for guidance and technical assistance on many matters pertaining to communicative disorders, including advice on such issues as (1) when should hearing-impaired persons be provided with rehabilitative assistance, (2) when should special services be provided to hearing-handicapped persons, (3) what constitutes a hearing handicap, and (4) when is a hearing handicap severe enough to warrant the payment of a disability award, financial assistance, or compensation for some injury or liability.

At times, the terms *hearing impairment, hearing handicap,* and *hearing disability* are used as if they are synonymous, when the terms should convey different meanings. In this report, these terms are defined in a manner similar to that advanced by the American Medical Association (1947, 1961, 1979). The term *hearing impairment* is used to mean a deviation or change for the worse in either auditory structure or auditory function, usually outside the range of normal. *Hearing handicap* means the disadvantage imposed by a hearing impairment on a person's communicative performance in the activities of daily living, and *hearing disability* means the determination of a financial award for the loss of function caused by any hearing impairment that results in significant hearing handicap.

*American Speech-Language-Hearing Association Task Force on the Definition of Hearing Handicap, 1980: *Members:* Louise Colodzin; Gene A. Del Polito; Donna M. Dickman; Alan S. Feldman (former member); Thomas G. Giolas; Robert M. McLauchlin; Roy Sullivan. *Consultants:* Edward Hardick; William Melnick; Alice Suter. Reprinted by permission.

### factors contributing to hearing handicap

Defining the parameters of hearing handicap is a very complex task since impaired hearing is itself a very complex phenomenon. Persons with conductive hearing problems do not experience the same kinds of communicative problems or manifestations of auditory dysfunction presented by persons with sensorineural hearing loss, and the communicative problems and auditory manifestations presented by persons with peripheral hearing problems are not the same as those presented by others with central auditory dysfunction. The degree to which a hearing impairment is a handicapping condition will depend on the interaction of a number of factors, and ideally any definition of hearing handicap should be based on a comprehensive consideration of the interrelationship of such factors as:

> the present age of the individual,
>
> the age of the individual when the impairment developed,
>
> the age of the person when the impairment was first discovered,
>
> the nature and extent of the hearing impairment,
>
> the person's communicative needs and the nature of the settings in which communication occurs,
>
> the relationship of the hearing impairment to other physical or mental impairments,
>
> the amount and success of rehabilitative treatment already received,
>
> the individual's reaction and the reaction of others to his or her impaired hearing, and
>
> the effect of the hearing impairment on the individual's expressive communicative ability.

Specialists in communicative disorders deal with these variables in a clinical setting on a daily basis. They often are asked to provide expert judgments of the extent and nature of individuals' hearing impairments and hearing handicaps. Indeed, the determination of hearing handicap *requires* the judgment of qualified professionals who possess the requisite expert knowledge of human communication and its disorders. Ideally, decisions to grant compensation or some other financial award for hearing disability should be based on a sound professional judgment of the nature and degree of the handicapping condition. The size of a hearing disability award should be in direct proportion to the extent of the hearing handicap, and the method used for determining hearing handicap should be capable of discerning relatively small differences between handicapping conditions. Optimally, all of the factors that contribute to making the hearing impairment a handicapping condition should be discretely quantified and interrelated in an unambiguous manner, so that even a relatively untrained individual would be able to arrive at a reasonable determination of hearing disability. Unfortunately, no means currently exist to quantify and interrelate these factors in a way that would meet with widespread professional agreement.

The task of defining hearing handicap is awesome, since the definition should apply to a variety of circumstances, e.g., determining when a preschool child or schoolchild requires rehabilitative or special education assistance, determining when a child or adult qualifies for supplemental security income benefits, determining when an adult requires comprehensive or vocational rehabilitative assistance, determining when a worker or accident victim deserves financial compensation for an acquired handicapping condition, and many others. Presently, no one definition of hearing handicap will adequately meet all the administrative or social program needs of hearing-impaired persons. Rather, it is necessary to define hearing handicap in a variety of ways to address the particular needs of society's health, education, and welfare programs. This report represents an attempt to address only one of those needs—a definition of hearing handicap useful in workers' compensation proceedings.

### hearing handicap and compensation

For many years, it has been recognized that engaging in certain noisy occupations for extended periods of time without adequate hearing protection can result in permanent changes in hearing function. Since the 1950s, the federal and state courts have maintained the liability of employers to compensate employees financially for hearing handicaps incurred as a result of job-related conditions (Newby 1964; Ginnold 1974; McLauchlin 1978; Ginnold 1979). The orderly and equitable payment of compensation for hearing handicap requires a means for determining not only the existence but also the extent of hearing handicap. Over the years, a number of pure tone and speech audiometric methods have been used for making this determination, including:

> the Fletcher 0.8 rule which was derived from loudness and intelligibility data reported by Fletcher (1929) as a means for assessing hearing loss for speech;
>
> the 1942 American Medical Association (AMA) formula for estimating percentage of hearing loss on the basis of percent values ascribed to hearing threshold data at octave intervals between 256 and 4095 Hz (AMA, 1942);
>
> the Fowler-Sabine, or AMA, method, which used a frequency-weighted average of hearing thresholds at 500, 1000, 2000, and 4000 Hz (AMA 1947);
>
> the 1959 American Academy of Ophthalmology and Otolaryngology (AAOO) formula, which used a simple average of hearing thresholds at 500, 1000, and 2000 Hz with a low fence and high fence cutoff for determining minimum and maximum impairment (AAOO 1959);

the Veterans Administration method (VA 1976) and the Social Adequacy Index (Davis 1948), which derived hearing handicap based on spondee thresholds and word discrimination test performance; and

questionnaires or self-evaluation techniques (Nett, Doerfler, and Matthews 1959; High, Fairbanks, and Glorig 1964; Noble and Atherly 1970; Alpiner 1978; Noble 1978; Giolas, Owens, Lamb, and Schubert 1979).

Of all these methods, the formula advanced by the American Academy of Ophthalmology and Otolaryngology (AAOO) in 1959 has been used most widely as a basis for judicial and administrative determination of hearing disability. The AAOO formula has been used in eighteen states as a means for determining workers' compensation awards, but has been criticized by the scientific community in recent years because (1) the formula's low fence for beginning handicap was too high and the high fence for establishing total handicap was too severe (Kryter 1970; Kryter 1973; Noble 1978; Suter 1978a; Ginnold 1979) and (2) the rule discounted the value of high-frequency hearing to understanding speech in everyday listening circumstances including noisy listening conditions (Kryter, Williams, and Green 1962; Niemeyer 1967; NIOSH 1972; Kuzniarz 1973; Anianson 1974; Burns 1977; Suter 1978a; Ginnold 1979). Consequently, some states—including California, New Jersey, and Wisconsin—have chosen not to use the 1959 AAOO formula for workers' compensation hearing disability claims because of one or more of the above criticisms. In 1969, the U.S. Department of Labor Office of Workers' Compensation Programs (OWCP) abandoned the use of the 1959 AAOO method and adopted a variant of the formula which used high frequency threshold data for the determination of hearing disability (GAO 1978).

Cognizant of the deficiencies that plagued the 1959 AAOO formula, the American Academy of Otolaryngology (AAO) recently revised its method for evaluating hearing handicap by incorporating hearing threshold data obtained at 3000 Hz as well as data from 500, 1000, and 2000 Hz (AMA 1979). Percent hearing handicap for each ear is predicted by averaging hearing thresholds at the four frequencies, subtracting 25 from the average, and multiplying the result by 1.5.

Throughout the United States, the determination of the point at which a hearing impairment becomes a hearing handicap and the point at which that hearing handicap becomes a hearing disability is based on a variety of approaches (Ginnold 1979). The lack of a generally accepted method for predicting hearing handicap has done little to assure that compensation awards granted under federal and state statutes are tempered by a meaningful reference to the degree of actual hearing handicap experienced by the individual. Discussions of methods for predicting hearing handicap at meetings of professional societies often turn into debates over the economic impact of one method or another on the financial awards granted to work-ers' compensation plaintiffs. Arguments of this type sap the vitality from the potential contributions those with expert knowledge might be able to ren-der for society. How much an individual receives as compensation for his or her occupationally related hearing loss is a value judgment that is dele-gated to a society's duly constituted authorities who are charged with mak-ing administrative and judicial decisions about disability and should not be a factor confounding a professional's judgment about the extent of a hear-ing handicap.

Conversely, deciding how to define and describe when a hearing impair-ment becomes a hearing handicap is not a decision that should be left to administrators and lawyers. These are decisions that should be made by those with the requisite expertise in assessing human communication and its disorders. It is here where professional societies and their members can make a meaningful contribution to the social welfare by applying their professional talents in an appropriate manner. In this regard, then, the following sets forth a proposed procedure and a rationale for predicting degree of hearing handicap in a format that might be suitable as a basis for determining hearing disability for workers' compensation.

### an alternate method for predicting hearing handicap

As stated earlier, the point at which a hearing impairment becomes a hearing handicap will depend on several factors that go beyond a simple statement of the degree of hearing loss (i.e., an individual's age, onset of the problem, communicative need, etc.). Ideally, a method of describing degree of hearing handicap should be based on a comprehensive consider-ation of all these factors. To be useful as a means for determining hearing disability, however, the definition of hearing handicap should be straightfor-ward and unambiguous, and hearing handicap judgments based on this definition should be consistent from one examiner to another. Unfortu-nately, there currently is no method of interrelating the variables that con-tribute to hearing handicap to produce uniformly consistent judgments regarding degree of hearing handicap across examiners.

There are many methods that can be used to assess hearing impairment; of them all, the methods for measuring pure tone auditory threshold sen-sitivity are very similar throughout the world. Tests of pure tone threshold sensitivity also can be administered using behavioral or electrophysiologic measurement techniques that can reduce the confounding influences of differences in listener sophistication or linguistic competence. On the other hand, there are no universally accepted or universally used measures of speech discrimination ability. While some speech discrimination measures, such as the CID Auditory Test W-22, enjoy more widespread use in the

United States than others, no one measure of speech discrimination ability will meet the needs of all examiners for use with all hearing-impaired persons. Some speech discrimination tests require greater test-taking sophistication, linguistic facility, and literacy from the listener than other tests. Additionally, methods for determining listener response reliability and accuracy in the presence of pseudohypocusis are not well developed for speech discrimination measures. Response reliability and accuracy also can vary markedly when the materials used are not presented in the listener's native language.

Claims for workers' compensation are made primarily by persons with occupational histories of prolonged exposure to high levels of noise. Noise-induced damage to peripheral auditory structures can result in fairly predictable patterns of threshold sensitivity loss, but delineating a method for predicting hearing handicap solely on the basis of pure tone threshold data must be done with caution. Such an approach is reasonable only if those who use it are fully aware of its shortcomings.

***Selection of Frequencies.*** Most everyday speech communication takes place under less-than-ideal listening circumstances (Pearson 1976; Harris 1965; Niemeyer 1967; Kryter 1973). Most human communication occurs in the presence of some degree of acoustic competition, and competing sounds will further degrade the intelligibility of speech received by hearing-impaired listeners. It is only reasonable to assume that any attempt to establish a relationship between pure tone sensitivity and speech discrimination ability should be done with speech discrimination data obtained under less-than-quiet listening conditions, since the objective of such a comparison is to determine when hearing impairment will disrupt communicative performance under conditions encountered in daily living.

A number of investigators have explored the relationship between threshold sensitivity and discrimination ability in quiet and in noise (Mullins and Banks 1956; Kryter, Williams, and Green 1962; Ross, Huntington, Newby, and Dixon 1965; Acton 1970; Elkins 1971; Lindeman 1971; Anianson 1974; Kuzniarz 1973; Dickman 1974) and have affirmed the importance of hearing sensitivity at 1000, 2000, 3000, and 4000 Hz for the discrimination of a variety of speech stimuli under quiet and noise listening conditions. Suter (1978a) noted that pure tone threshold data at 500, 1000, and 2000 Hz were the poorest predictors of speech discrimination ability in quiet or in noise; and when a variety of frequency combinations were examined, averaged threshold information at 1000, 2000, and 4000 Hz best predicted listener performance in noise. Suter concluded that any technique for assessing the ability of hearing-impaired individuals to understand speech in everyday listening conditions must include information regarding hearing above 2000 Hz.

*Establishing the Low and High Fences* To be useful, any method used to describe the degree of hearing handicap on the basis of pure tone data (1) must define the threshold of beginning hearing handicap (the low fence), (2) must define the point at which a hearing impairment results in what must be considered a very severe, or complete, hearing handicap (the high fence), and (3) must provide a means for describing the degree of hearing handicap between these two extremes. Just as there are a variety of approaches for defining hearing handicap, there are almost as many approaches for describing or setting the low and high fences for hearing handicap.

For instance, in the Fletcher method, or the 0.8 rule, the range of hearing for the average of hearing thresholds at 500, 1000, and 2000 Hz was divided into degrees of hearing loss from 0 dB to 120 dB SPL (Fletcher 1929). In the Fowler-Sabine or AMA method (AMA 1947) percentage hearing handicap values were determined by differentially weighting pure tone thresholds at 500, 1000, 2000, and 4000 Hz. A threshold for hearing handicap was established at 20 dB HL (ANSI 1969) and a ceiling was set at 105 dB HL (ANSI 1969). Hearing handicap is assessed by the Veterans Administration using spondee thresholds, monosyllabic speech discrimination scores, and pure tone thresholds at 250, 500, 1000, 2000, and 4000 Hz (VA 1976). The veteran's hearing is considered normal if spondee thresholds are less than 26 dB HL (ANSI 1969), if discrimination scores are above 92% in each ear, and if all pure tone thresholds between 250 and 4000 Hz are less than 40 dB HL and less than 25 dB HL for at least four frequencies. Maximum handicap is defined, generally, as when spondee thresholds exceed 96 dB HL regardless of speech discrimination ability or when speech discrimination ability is less than 40% regardless of spondee threshold level. In the 1959 AAOO method, no hearing handicap (i.e., the low fence) is said to exist when the average of hearing thresholds at 500, 1000, and 2000 Hz is 25 dB HL (ANSI 1969) or better. Complete hearing handicap (i.e., the high fence) is defined as an average of hearing thresholds at 500, 1000, and 2000 Hz of 92 dB HL (ANSI 1969) or more.

There have been other approaches to defining low fence and high fence values, but they are basically only variations of the 1959 AAOO approach. For instance, in California the 25 dB low fence and the 92 dB high fence from the AAOO formula have been retained, but the frequencies used to calculate the frequency average are 500, 1000, 2000, and 3000 Hz instead of only 500, 1000, and 2000 Hz. This approach is identical to that which was adopted by the AMA in its most recent (1979) revision. Similarly, the U.S. Department of Labor Office of Workers' Compensation Programs also retained the 1959 AAOO low and high fence dB values, but calculated the hearing frequency average using threshold information at 1000, 2000, and 3000 Hz instead of 500, 1000, and 2000 Hz. The Committee on Hearing, Bioacoustics, and Biomechanism of the National Academy of Sciences

(CHABA) has offered yet another alternate approach based on a simple average of hearing thresholds at 1000, 2000, and 3000 Hz by setting the low fence at 35 dB (CHABA 1975). The purpose of CHABA's exercise, however, was to determine a low fence using 1000, 2000, and 3000 Hz that would result in no additional compensation than if a 25 dB low fence were used with an average of hearing thresholds at 500, 1000, and 2000 Hz.

Kryter (1973) has argued that the 1959 AAOO 25 dB low fence value was too high since it failed to account for when communication occurred in the presence of background noise. Kryter predicted that an individual with a hearing level of 25 dB at 500, 1000, and 2000 Hz would be able to repeat correctly only 90% of sentence test items at a normal conversational intensity level. He argued that if hearing thresholds at 500, 1000, and 2000 Hz are to be used for determining degree of hearing handicap, then the low fence should be set at 15 dB HL (ANSI 1969) and not at 25 dB HL. Similarly, Kryter felt that the 1959 AAOO high fence of 92 dB HL (ANSI) was unrealistic. He argued that the point at which most listeners would no longer be able to understand speech at everyday conversational levels was considerably lower than 92 dB. Kryter proposed setting the high fence at 75 dB when based on the average of hearing thresholds at 1000, 2000, and 3000 Hz.

Suter (1978a) compared her data on the performance of normal and hearing-impaired listeners on speech discrimination measures with data reported by Acton (1970). She noted that a 25 dB low fence was too high even when hearing thresholds were averaged at 1000, 2000, and 3000 Hz. She argued that when speech discrimination testing was performed in the presence of background noise, a low fence that would differentiate between handicapped and nonhandicapped persons would be more appropriate if set at 10 dB HL (ANSI 1969) when averaging pure tone thresholds at 1000, 2000, and 3000 HZ and at 22 dB HL (ANSI 1969) when averaging over thresholds at 1000, 2000, and 4000 Hz.

The low fence and high fence values used in any hearing handicap determination should be set in some reasonable relationship to the degree of communicative difficulty hearing-impaired individuals actually experience. The low fence should be set at a value above which it is reasonable to assume that hearing handicap exists, while the high fence should be set at a value above which it is reasonable to assume that the hearing handicap is complete. In this context, then, there is a reasonable certainty that a hearing-impaired adult would experience some degree of difficulty in discriminating speech under everyday listening conditions when the average of hearing thresholds at 1000, 2000, 3000, and 4000 Hz is poorer than 25 dB HL (the low fence). Furthermore, when an individual's average of hearing thresholds at 1000, 2000, 3000, and 4000 Hz exceeds 75 dB HL (the high fence), hearing handicap essentially can be considered complete, since conservation would be difficult to sustain for more than only short periods of time because a speaker would have to exert excessive vocal effort in order to communicate. Even at sustained intensity levels, the ability of such a severely hearing-impaired person to discriminate the high-frequency acoustic cues necessary for the understanding of speech would be minimal.

*Growth of Handicap* The simplest means for describing the growth of hearing handicap between these two extremes (i.e., 25 dB low fence and 75 dB high fence) is to assume a linear growth pattern of 2% for each dB increase in averaged hearing loss above 25 dB. While the actual growth in hearing handicap over this range may not be described perfectly by a linear function, using a nonlinear growth pattern for determining degree of hearing handicap would be cumbersome. In a subsequent analysis of her own data obtained from hearing-impaired listeners on speech discrimination tasks conducted in the presence of acoustic competition, Suter (1978b) reported that the relationship between listener speech discrimination performance and average listener hearing level at 1000, 2000, and 4000 Hz was described best by a linear function. Consequently, the assumption of a linear growth in hearing handicap over the range of average hearing levels at 1000, 2000, 3000, and 4000 Hz between 25 dB and 75 dB appears to be reasonable. Using a 2% linear growth rate simplifies even further the computation of predicted percent handicap compared to the 1.5% linear growth rate used in the AAOO (1959) and AMA (1979) formulae.

*Unique Characteristic of This Alternate Approach* This approach for predicting hearing handicap differs from previous methods in that it discounts hearing loss greater than 75 dB when calculating the average amount of hearing loss across the four frequencies. For instance, if an individual's hearing threshold sensitivity at 1000, 2000, 3000, and 4000 Hz were 60 dB, 75 dB, 85 dB, and 90 dB, the figures used to calculate the average hearing loss across the four frequencies would be 60 dB, 75 dB, 75 dB, and 75 dB. A hearing loss of 75 dB effectively precludes an individual from hearing the higher-frequency formants and formant transitions essential to understanding everyday speech without the assistance of electronic amplification. The degree of handicap experienced by the unaided listener would be no more complete when thresholds at or above 1000 Hz exceeded 75 dB, and little is gained by accounting for the additional hearing loss above 75 dB when calculating the degree of hearing handicap.

*Weighting the Importance of the Two Ears* Currently, there are no known data to support or refute the method used by the AMA for calculating predicted percent binaural handicap. Investigations should be encouraged to determine the validity of using specific better ear/poorer ear weighting procedures to determine binaural hearing handicap. In the meantime, a 5:1 better ear/poorer ear weighting applied to the calculation of binaural hearing handicap will suffice.

## summary

In this report, the terms *hearing impairment, hearing handicap,* and *hearing disability* have been used to signify distinct ideas. *Hearing impairment* is defined as a deviation or change for the worse in either auditory structure or auditory function, usually outside the range of normal. *Hearing handicap* means the disadvantage imposed by a hearing impairment on a person's performance in the activities of daily living. *Hearing disability* means the determination of a financial award for the actual or presumed loss of ability to perform activities of daily living.

Hearing impairment, particularly hearing sensitivity, is easily quantifiable using procedures that are widely accepted within the professional community. Hearing handicap, however, is much more difficult to determine—so often hearing handicap is predicted on the basis of measures of hearing sensitivity. The problem with this predictive process is that many factors other than hearing sensitivity contribute to hearing handicap. While experimental efforts to quantify and interrelate these other contributing factors to hearing handicap should be encouraged in order to improve the accuracy of determining hearing handicap, the use of measures of hearing sensitivity as a means for determining hearing handicap should not be abandoned. In this report, a proposed method for determining degree of hearing handicap for workers' compensation purposes has been set forth. The method differs from others in that degree of hearing handicap is determined by:

averaging hearing thresholds at 1000, 2000, 3000, and 4000 Hz;

setting a low fence of 25 dB and a high fence of 75 dB;

disregarding additional hearing sensitivity loss above 75 dB at the form frequencies used to calculate average hearing threshold level;

assuming a 2%/dB linear growth of hearing handicap between the 25 dB low fence and the 75 dB high fence.

## references

ACTON, W. I. Speech intelligibility in a background noise and noise-induced hearing loss. *Ergonomics* 13: 546–554 (1970).

ALPINER, J. G., ed. *Handbook of adult rehabilitative audiology.* Appendix 3D, The Denver Scale of Communication Function. Baltimore: Williams & Wilkins (1978).

AMERICAN ACADEMY OF OPHTHALMOLOGY AND OTOLARYNGOLOGY COMMITTEE ON CONSERVATION OF HEARING. Guide for the evaluation of hearing impairment. *Trans. Am. Acad. Ophthalmol. Otolaryngol.* 63: 236–238 (1959).

AMERICAN MEDICAL ASSOCIATION COUNCIL ON PHYSICAL THERAPY. Tentative standard procedure for evaluating the percentage loss of hearing in medicolegal cases. *J. Amer. Med. Assn.* 19: 1108–1109 (1942).

AMERICAN MEDICAL ASSOCIATION COUNCIL ON PHYSICAL MEDICINE. Tentative standard procedure for evaluating the percentage loss of hearing in medicolegal cases. *J. Amer. Med. Assn.* 133: 396–397 (1947).

AMERICAN MEDICAL ASSOCIATION COMMITTEE ON MEDICAL RATING OF PHYSICAL IMPAIRMENT. Guide to the evaluation of permanent impairment: ear, nose, throat, and related structures. *J. Amer. Med. Assn.* 177: 489–501 (1961).

AMERICAN MEDICAL ASSOCIATION. Guide for the evaluation of hearing handicap. *J. Amer. Med. Assn.* 241: 2055–2059 (1979).

AMERICAN NATIONAL STANDARDS INSTITUTE. *Specifications for Audiometers.* ANSI S3.6–1969 (R1973). New York: Acoustical Society of America (1973).

ANIANSON, G. Methods for assessing high frequency hearing loss in everyday listening situations. *Acta. Otol.* Suppl. 320 (1974).

BURNS, W. Comments on industrial deafness review. Unpublished report (1977).

DAVIS, H. The articulation area and the Social Adequacy Index for hearing. *Laryngoscope* 58: 761–778 (1948).

FLETCHER, H. *Speech and hearing.* New York: Van Nostrand (1929).

GINNOLD, R. Workmen's compensation for hearing loss in Wisconsin. *Labor Law J.* 682–697 (1974).

GINNOLD, R. Workers' compensation for hearing loss: a review of state and federal programs. Unpublished draft report (1979).

GIOLAS, T. G., OWENS, E., LAMB, S., and SCHUBERT, E. Hearing performance inventory. *J. Speech Hearing Dis.* 44: 2 169–195 (1979).

HARRIS, J. D. Pure tone acuity and the intelligibility of everyday speech. *J. Acoust. Soc. Amer.* 37: 824–830 (1965).

HIGH, W. S., FAIRBANKS, G., and GLORIG, A. Scale for self-assessment of hearing handicap. *J. Speech Hearing Dis.* 29: 215–230 (1964).

KRYTER, K. D. *The effects of noise on man.* New York: Academic Press (1970).

KRYTER, K. D. Impairment to hearing from exposure to noise. *J. Acoust. Soc. Amer.* 53: 1211–1234 (1973).

KRYTER, K. D., WILLIAMS, C., and GREEN, D. M. Auditory acuity and the perception of speech. *J. Acoust. Soc. Amer.* 34: 1217–1223 (1962).

KUZNIARZ, J. J. Hearing loss and speech intelligibility in noise. In *Proceedings of the International Congress on Noise as a Public Health Problem.* U. S. Environmental Protection Administration Report 550/9-73-008 (1973).

LING, D. Rehabilitation of cases with deafness secondary to otitis media. In *Otitis Media,* ed. A. Glorig and K. S. Gerwin, pp. 249–253. Springfield, Ill.: Charles C Thomas (1972).

McLAUCHLIN, R. M. Audiologists in the United States. In D. M. Lipscomb, Ed., *Noise and Audiology.* Baltimore: University Park Press (1978).

NATIONAL ACADEMY OF SCIENCES COMMITTEE ON HEARING, BIOACOUSTICS, AND BIOMECHANICS (CHABA) *Compensation formula for hearing loss.* Report of Working Group 77. Washington: National Academy of Sciences (1975).

NETT, E. M., DOERFLER, L. G., and MATTHEWS, J. The relationship between audiological measures and handicap. Unpublished report, University of Pittsburgh School of Medicine (1959).

NEWBY, H. A. *Audiology.* 2nd ed. Englewood Cliffs, New Jersey: Prentice-Hall, Inc. (1964).

NORTHERN, J. L. and DOWNS, M. P. *Hearing in children.* 2nd ed. Baltimore: Williams & Wilkins (1978).

NIEMEYER, W. Speech discrimination in noise-induced deafness. International Audiology 6: 42–47 (1967).

NOBLE, W. G. and ATHERLY, G. R. C. The hearing measurement scale. *J. Aud. Res.* 10: 229–250 (1970).

NOBLE, W. G. *Assessment of impaired hearing: a critique and new method.* New York: Academic Press (1978).

PEARSONS, K. S., BENNETT, R. L., and FIDELL, S. *Speech levels in various environments.* BBN Report No. 3281.: Bolt, Beranek, and Newman (1976).

SUTER, A. H. *The ability of mildly hearing-impaired individuals to discriminate speech in noise.* U.S. Environmental Protection Administration Report 550/9-78-100 AMRL-TR-78-4 (1978a).

SUTER, A. H. Personal communication (1978b).

U.S. DEPARTMENT OF HEALTH, EDUCATION, AND WELFARE NATIONAL INSTITUTE FOR OCCUPATIONAL SAFETY AND HEALTH (NIOSH). *Criteria for a recommended standard: occupational exposure to noise.* HSM 73–1001 (1972).

U.S. GENERAL ACCOUNTING OFFICE (GAO). *To provide proper compensation for hearing impairments, the Labor Department should change its criteria.* Report to the Congress of the United States by the Comptroller General (1978).

U.S. VETERANS ADMINISTRATION (VA). *Rating procedure relative to specific issues: 50.07 rating of hearing impairment.* Department of Medicine and Surgery Manual, M21-1 (1976).

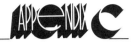

○ HEARING HANDICAP SCALE*

### form A

1. If you are six to twelve feet from the loudspeaker of a radio do you understand speech well?
2. Can you carry on a telephone conversation without difficulty?
3. If you are six to twelve feet away from a television set, do you understand most of what is said?
4. Can you carry on a conversation with one other person when you are on a noisy street corner?
5. Do you hear all right when you are in a street car, airplane, bus, or train?
6. If there are noises from other voices, typewriters, traffic, music, etc., can you understand when someone speaks to you?
7. Can you understand a person when you are seated beside him and cannot see his face?
8. Can you understand if someone speaks to you while you are chewing crisp foods, such as potato chips or celery?
9. Can you carry on a conversation with one other person when you are in a noisy place, such as a restaurant or at a party?
10. Can you understand if someone speaks to you in a whisper and you can't see his face?
11. When you talk with a bus driver, waiter, ticket salesman, etc., can you understand all right?
12. Can you carry on a conversation if you are seated across the room from someone who speaks in a normal tone of voice?
13. Can you understand women when they talk?
14. Can you carry on a conversation with one other person when you are out of doors and it is reasonably quiet?
15. When you are in a meeting or at a large dinner table, would you know the speaker was talking if you could not see his lips moving?
16. Can you follow the conversation when you are at a large dinner table or in a meeting with a small group?
17. If you are seated under the balcony of a theater or auditorium, can you hear well enough to follow what is going on?

*W. S. High, G. Fairbanks, and A. Glorig, "Scale of Self-Assessment of Hearing Handicap," *Journal of Speech and Hearing Disorders,* 29 (1964), pp. 215–230. Reprinted by permission.

18. When you are in a large formal gathering (a church, lodge, lecture hall, etc.) can you hear what is said when the speaker *does not* use a microphone?

19. Can you hear the telephone ring when you are in the room where it is located?

20. Can you hear warning signals, such as automobile horns, railway crossing bells, or emergency vehicle sirens?

### form B

1. When you are listening to the radio or watching television, can you hear adequately when the volume is comfortable for most other people?

2. Can you carry on a conversation with one other person when you are riding in an automobile with the windows *closed?*

3. Can you carry on a conversation with one other person when you are riding in an automobile with the window *open?*

4. Can you carry on a conversation with one other person if there is a radio or television in the same room playing at normal loudness?

5. Can you hear when someone calls to you from another room?

6. Can you understand when someone speaks to you from another room?

7. When you buy something in a store, do you easily understand the clerk?

8. Can you carry on a conversation with someone who does not speak as loudly as most people?

9. Can you tell if a person is talking when you are seated beside him and cannot see his face?

10. When you ask someone for directions, do you understand what he says?

11. If you are within three or four feet of a person who speaks in a normal tone of voice (assume you are facing one another), can you hear everything he says?

12. Do you recognize the voices of speakers when you don't see them?

13. When you are introduced to someone, can you understand the name the first time it is spoken?

14. Can you hear adequately when you are conversing with more than one person?

15. If you are in an audience, such as in a church or theatre and you are seated near the *front,* can you understand most of what is said?

16. Can you carry on everyday conversations with members of your family without difficulty?

17. If you are in an audience, such as in a church or theatre and you are seated near the *rear,* can you understand most of what is said?

18. When you are in a large formal gathering (a church, lodge, lecture hall, etc.) can you hear what is said when the speaker *does* use a microphone?

19. Can you hear the telephone ring when you are in the next room?

20. Can you hear night sounds, such as distant trains, bells, dogs barking, trucks passing, and so forth?

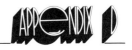

○ THE DENVER SCALE OF COMMUNICATION FUNCTION*

Pre-Service_____     Post-Service_____

Date _____     Case No. _____

Name _____Age ___Sex___

Address _____

        (City)          (State)         (Zip)

Lives Alone_____In Apartment _____Retired_____
                     (if no, specify)

Occupation _____

Audiogram (Examination Date_____Agency_____ )
  Pure Tone:

| | 250 | 500 | 1000 | 2000 | 4000 | 8000 | Hz |
|---|---|---|---|---|---|---|---|
| RE | — | — | — | — | — | — | |
| | | | | | | | dB (re: ANSI) |
| LE | — | — | — | — | — | — | |

Speech:

SRT           DISCRIMINATION SCORE (%)

                Quiet       Noise (S/N =   )

RE_____dB     RE_____

LE_____dB     LE_____

---

*Reproduced by permission from J. G. Alpiner, W. Chevrette, G. Glascoe, M. Metz, and B. Olsen. Unpublished Study, The University of Denver, © 1974.

Hearing Aid Information

Aided____For How Long_____Aid Type_____

Satisfaction _____


EXAMINER:_____


The following questionnaire was designed to evaluate your communication ability as you view it. You are asked to judge or scale each statement in the following manner.

If you judge the statement to be *very closely related* to either extreme, please place your check mark as follows:

Agree __X__  _____  _____  _____  _____  _____  _____ Disagree

or

Agree _____  _____  _____  _____  _____  _____  __X__ Disagree

If you judge the stagement to be *closely related* to either end of the scale, please mark as follows:

Agree _____  __X__  _____  _____  _____  _____  _____ Disagree

or

Agree _____  _____  _____  _____  _____  __X__  _____ Disagree

If you judge the statement to be only slightly related to either end of the scale, please mark as follows:

Agree _____  _____  __X__  _____  _____  _____  _____ Disagree

or

Agree _____  _____  _____  _____  __X__  _____  _____ Disagree

If you consider the statement to be irrelevant or unassociated to your communication situation, please mark as follows:

Agree _____  _____  _____  __X__  _____  _____  _____ Disagree

PLEASE NOTE:  Check a scale for every statement.

Put only one checkmark on each scale.

Make a separate judgment for each statement.

ALSO: You may comment on each statement in the space provided.


1. The members of my family are annoyed with my loss of hearing.
   Agree _____  _____  _____  _____  _____  _____  _____ Disagree
   Comments:
2. The members of my family sometimes leave me out of conversations or discussions.

Agree _____   _____   _____   _____   _____   _____   _____ Disagree
Comments:

3. Sometimes my family makes decisions for me because I have a hard time following discussions.
Agree _____   _____   _____   _____   _____   _____   _____ Disagree
Comments:

4. My family becomes annoyed when I ask them to repeat what was said because I did not hear them.
Agree _____   _____   _____   _____   _____   _____   _____ Disagree
Comments:

5. I am not an "outgoing" person because I have a hearing loss.
Agree _____   _____   _____   _____   _____   _____   _____ Disagree
Comments:

6. I now take less of an interest in many things as compared to when I did not have a hearing problem.
Agree _____   _____   _____   _____   _____   _____   _____ Disagree
Comments:

7. Other people do not realize how frustrated I get when I cannot hear or understand.
Agree _____   _____   _____   _____   _____   _____   _____ Disagree
Comments:

8. People sometimes avoid me because of my hearing loss.
Agree _____   _____   _____   _____   _____   _____   _____ Disagree
Comments:

9. I am not a calm person because of my hearing loss.
Agree _____   _____   _____   _____   _____   _____   _____ Disagree
Comments:

10. I tend to be negative about life in general because of my hearing loss.
Agree _____   _____   _____   _____   _____   _____   _____ Disagree
Comments:

11. I do not socialize as much as I did before I began to lose my hearing.
Agree _____   _____   _____   _____   _____   _____   _____ Disagree
Comments:

12. Since I have trouble hearing, I do not like to go places with friends.
Agree _____   _____   _____   _____   _____   _____   _____ Disagree
Comments:

13. Since I have trouble hearing, I hestitate to meet new people.
Agree _____   _____   _____   _____   _____   _____   _____ Disagree
Comments:

14. I do not enjoy my job as much as I did before I began to lose my hearing.
Agree _____   _____   _____   _____   _____   _____   _____ Disagree
Comments:

15. Other people do not understand what it is like to have a hearing loss.
Agree _____   _____   _____   _____   _____   _____   _____ Disagree
Comments:

16. Because I have difficulty understanding what is said to me, I sometimes answer questions wrong.
    Agree _____  _____  _____  _____  _____  _____  _____ Disagree
    Comments:
17. I do not feel relaxed in a communicative situation.
    Agree _____  _____  _____  _____  _____  _____  _____ Disagree
    Comments:
18. I do not feel comfortable in most communication situations.
    Agree _____  _____  _____  _____  _____  _____  _____ Disagree
    Comments:
19. Conversations in a noisy room prevent me from attempting to communicate with others.
    Agree _____  _____  _____  _____  _____  _____  _____ Disagree
    Comments:
20. I am not comfortable having to speak in a group situation.
    Agree _____  _____  _____  _____  _____  _____  _____ Disagree
    Comments:
21. In general, I do not find listening relaxing.
    Agree _____  _____  _____  _____  _____  _____  _____ Disagree
    Comments:
22. I feel threatened by many communication situations due to difficulty hearing.
    Agree _____  _____  _____  _____  _____  _____  _____ Disagree
    Comments:
23. I seldom watch other people's facial expressions when talking to them.
    Agree _____  _____  _____  _____  _____  _____  _____ Disagree
    Comments:
24. I hesitate to ask people to repeat if I do not understand them the first time they speak.
    Agree _____  _____  _____  _____  _____  _____  _____ Disagree
    Comments:
25. Because I have difficulty understanding what is said to me, I sometimes make comments that do not fit into the conversation.
    Agree _____  _____  _____  _____  _____  _____  _____ Disagree
    Comments:

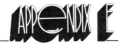

## ○ OBSERVATIONS FROM HEARING PERFORMANCE INVENTORY, EXPERIMENTAL FORM I

1. Female voices were consistently judged as harder to hear and understand.

2. There was a difference between all three noise environments with respondents indicating increasing difficulty in the following order: (1) quiet, (2) music or a crowd of people, and (3) people talking nearby.

3. No significant differences (less than a 0.20 SE) in reported communication difficulty were found between items in which the talker was spouse, family member, or friend. Such otherwise identical items were collapsed into one item with one talker, designated as *family member or friend.*

4. Significant differences between stranger as talker and the above three talkers were found only in noisy and other difficult listening situations (multiple talkers, etc.). Therefore, stranger items were retained only in these situations.

5. No significant differences were found between the items assessing talker distances of six of twelve feet. The twelve feet items were omitted.

6. Responses indicated consistently poorer performance for items describing conditions without visual cues than for the comparable listening conditions with visual cues. At the same time, no significant differences in communication difficulty were reported between listening to the radio and watching television.

7. As the listening conditions became more difficult (that is, with noise, multiple talkers, or no knowledge of the subject), responses indicated poorer performance, a wider distribution of responses, and sometimes a bimodal distribution of responses.

8. The *Response to Auditory Failure* section items showed sufficient variability, as evidenced by item standard deviations, to support the notion that respondents were not giving what they might think were approved responses.

9. Only 3% of the responses were omissions. The *Does not apply* response similarly was not used very often, actually accounting for less than 10% of the total responses and occurring mostly in the four hearing aid questions and the occupational items. For this reason the occupational items were placed at the end of the inventory as an optional section.

10. Approximately two-thirds of a set of items originally labelled *Personal* produced highly skewed distributions (in the direction of no difficulty) and thus did not differentiate the respondents from persons with no hearing difficulty. Accordingly, they were eliminated. The other third were retained and will be discussed later.

11. Sixty persons with normal hearing who acted as controls consistently marked the *No difficulty* (number 1) responses.

12. Fourteen items were repeated at random in the inventory for a consistency check. The average item reliability was 0.75 so, with reliability established, these duplicates were eliminated.

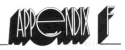

APPENDIX F

○ HEARING PERFORMANCE INVENTORY, FORM II
Thomas G. Giolas, University of Connecticut; Elmer Owens,
University of California; Stanford H. Lamb, San Francisco State
University; Earl D. Schubert, Stanford University

### instructions

We are interested in knowing how your hearing problem has affected your daily living. Below you will find a series of questions which describe a variety of everyday listening situations and ask you to judge how much difficulty you would have hearing in these situations. Once we know which situations cause a person difficulty, we can begin to do something about them. Your answers will be confidential.

The questions cover many different listening situations. Some ask you to judge how well you can understand what people are saying when their voices are loud enough. The term *understand* means hearing the words a person is saying clearly enough to be able to participate in the conversation. Other questions ask whether you can hear enough of a particular sound (doorbell, speech, etc.) to be aware of its presence. Other questions concern occupational, social, or personal situations. Still others ask what you *do* when you miss something that was said.

To answer each question, you are asked to check the phrase that best describes how often you experience the situation being described:

Practically always . . . . . . . . . . . . . . . . . . . . . . . . . . . . . . . . (or always)

Frequently . . . . . . . . . . . . . . . . . . . . (about three-quarters of the time)

About half the time

Occasionally . . . . . . . . . . . . . . . . . . . . . (about a quarter of the time)

Almost never . . . . . . . . . . . . . . . . . . . . . . . . . . . . . . . . . . (or never)

For example, if you can understand what a person is saying on the telephone about 100% of the time, then you should check *practically always*. On the other hand, if you can understand almost nothing of what a person is saying on the telephone, then you should check *almost never*. If you can understand what a person is saying on the telephone about 50% of the

173

time, then you should check *about half the time.*

Your answers to the questions should describe your hearing ability as it is now. If you wear a hearing aid in the situation described, answer the question accordingly. Please check *one, and only one,* phrase for each question. You should check *does not apply* only if you have not experienced a particular situation or one similar to it.

There are also questions that appear identical but differ in at least one important detail. Please read each question carefully before checking the appropriate phrase.

We know that all people do not talk alike. Some mumble, others talk too fast, and others talk without moving their lips very much. Please answer the questions according to the way *most* people talk to you.

If the question does not specify whether the person speaking is male or female, answer according to which sex you have the most difficulty hearing.

Asterisks on the score sheet are for scoring purposes and should be ignored.

1. You are with a male friend or family member in a fairly quiet room. Can you understand him when his voice is loud enough for you and you can see his face?

2. You are with a female friend or family member in a fairly quiet room. Can you understand her when her voice is loud enough for you and you can see her face?

3. You are with a female stranger in a fairly quiet room. Can you understand her when her voice is loud enough for you and you can see her face?

4. You are with a male stranger in a fairly quiet room. Can you understand him when his voice is loud enough for you and you can see his face?

5. You are with a child (6 to 10 years old) in a fairly quiet room. Can you understand the child when his/her voice is loud enough for you and you can see his/her face?

6. You are at a fairly quiet restaurant. Can you understand the waiter/waitress when his/her voice is loud enough for you and you can see his/her face?

7. You are at a restaurant with a friend or family member and the room is fairly quiet. Can you understand the person when his/her voice is loud enough for you and you can see his/her face?

8. You are in a fairly quiet room. Can you carry on a conversation with a man in another room if his voice is loud enough for you?

9. You are in a fairly quiet room. Can you carry on a conversation with a woman in another room if her voice is loud enough for you?

10. You are at a party or gathering of less than ten people and the room is fairly quiet. Can you understand what a friend or family member is saying to you when his/her voice is loud enough for you and you can see his/her face?

11. You are playing cards, monopoly, or some similar game with several people and the room is fairly quiet. Can you understand what a friend or family member is saying to you when his/her voice is loud enough for you and you can see his/her face?

12. You are in a fairly quiet room with five or six friends or family members. One person talks at a time. When you are aware of the subject, can you understand what is being said when the speaker's voice is loud enough for you and you can see his/her face?

13. You are in a fairly quiet room talking with five or six strangers. One person talks at a time and the subject of conversation changes from time to time. Can you understand what is being said when the speaker's voice is loud enough for you and you can see his/her face?

14. You are watching your favorite news program on television. Can you understand the news reporter (male) when his voice is loud enough for you?

15. You are watching your favorite news program on television. Can you understand the news reporter (female) when her voice is loud enough for you?

16. You are watching a drama or movie on television. Can you understand what is being said when the speaker's voice is loud enough for you and there is *no* music in the background?

17. You are watching a drama or movie on television. Can you understand what is being said when the speaker's voice is loud enough for you and there *is* music in the background?

18. You are in an auditorium listening to a lecturer (male) who is using a microphone. Can you understand what he is saying when his voice is loud enough for you and you can see his face?

19. You are in an auditorium listening to a lecturer (female) who is using a microphone. Can you understand what she is saying when her voice is loud enough for you and you can see her face?

20. When an announcement is given over a public-address system in a bus station or airport, can you understand what is being said when the speaker's voice is loud enough for you?

21. Can you understand what a man is saying on the telephone when his voice is loud enough for you?

22. Can you understand what a woman is saying on the telephone when her voice is loud enough for you?

23. You are at a movie. Can you understand what the actors/actresses are saying when their voices are loud enough for you and you can see their faces?

24. You are attending a stage play. Can you understand what the actors/actresses are saying when their voices are loud enough for you and you can see their faces?

25. You are with a male friend or family member and several people are talking nearby. Can you understand him when his voice is loud enough for you and you can see his face?

26. You are with a female friend or family member and several people are talking nearby. Can you understand her when her voice is loud enough for you and you can see her face?

27. You are with a female friend or family member and there is background noise such as traffic, music, or a crowd of people. Can you understand her when her voice is loud enough for you and you can see her face?

28. You are with a male stranger and there is background noise such as traffic, music, or a crowd of people. Can you understand him when his voice is loud enough for you and you can see his face?

29. You are with a female stranger and there is background noise such as traffic, music, or a crowd of people. Can you understand her when her voice is loud enough for you and you can see her face?

30. You are with a child (6 to 10 years old) and several people are talking nearby. Can you understand the child when his/her voice is loud enough for you and you can see his/her face?

31. You are with a child (6 to 10 years old) and there is background noise such as traffic, music, or a crowd of people. Can you understand the child when his/her voice is loud enough for you and you can see his/her face?

32. You are at a restaurant and several people are talking nearby. Can you understand the waiter/waitress when his/her voice is loud enough for you and you can see his/her face?

33. You are at a restaurant and there is background noise such as music or a crowd of people. Can you understand the waiter/waitress when his/her voice is loud enough for you and you can see his/her face?

34. You are at a restaurant with a friend or family member and several people are talking nearby. Can you understand the person when his/her voice is loud enough for you and you can see his/her face?

35. You are at a restaurant with a friend or family member and there is background noise such as music or a crowd of people. Can you understand the person when his/her voice is loud enough for you and you can see his/her face?

36. You are at a party or gathering of less than ten people and several people are talking nearby. Can you understand what a friend or family member (male) is saying to you when his voice is loud enough for you and you can see his face?

37. You are at a party or gathering of less than ten people and several people are talking nearby. Can you understand what a friend or family member (female) is saying to you when her voice is loud enough for you and you can see her face?

38. You are at a party or gathering of more than twenty people and several people are talking nearby. Can you understand what a friend or family member (female) is saying to you when her voice is loud enough for you and you can see her face?

39. You are at a party or gathering of more than twenty people and several people are talking nearby. Can you understand what a friend or family member (male) is saying to you when his voice is loud enough for you and you can see his face?

40. You are at a party or gathering of more than twenty people and there is background noise such as music or a crowd of people. Can you understand

what a stranger is saying to you when his/her voice is loud enough for you and you can see his/her face?

41. You are playing cards, monopoly, or some similar game with several people and other people are talking nearby. Can you understand what a friend or family member is saying to you when his/her voice is loud enough for you and you can see his/her face?

42. You are playing cards, monopoly, or some similar game with several people and there is background noise such as music or a crowd of people. Can you understand what a friend or family member is saying to you when his/her voice is loud enough for you and you can see his/her face?

43. You are with five or six friends or family members at a gathering of more than twenty people and there is background noise such as music or a crowd of people. One person talks at a time. When you are aware of the subject, can you understand what is being said when the speaker's voice is loud enough for you and you can see his/her face?

44. You are with five or six strangers at a gathering of more than twenty people and there is background noise such as music or a crowd of people. One person talks at a time. When you are aware of the subject, can you understand what is being said when the speaker's voice is loud enough for you and you can see his/her face?

45. You are with five or six friends or family members at a gathering of more than twenty people and several people are talking nearby. One person talks at a time and the subject of conversation changes from time to time. Can you understand what is being said when the speaker's voice is loud enough for you and you can see his/her face?

46. You are with five or six friends or family members at a gathering of more than twenty people and there is background noise such as music or a crowd of people. One person talks at a time and the subject of conversation changes from time to time. Can you understand what is being said when the speaker's voice is loud enough for you and you can see his/her face?

47. You are having dinner with five or six friends or family members at home and there is background noise such as music or a crowd of people. Can you understand what is being said when the speaker's voice is loud enough for you and you can see his/her face?

48. You are seated with five or six strangers around a table or in a living room. Often two persons are talking at once and one person frequently interrupts another. Can you understand what is being said when the speaker's voice is loud enough for you and you can see his/her face?

49. You are playing cards, monopoly, or some similar game and several people are talking nearby. The subject of conversation changes from time to time. Can you understand what is being said when the speaker's voice is loud enough for you and you can see his/her face?

50. You are riding in an automobile with several friends or family members. The windows are *closed* and you are sitting in the front seat. Can you understand the driver when his/her voice is loud enough for you and you can see his/her face?

51. You are riding in an automobile with several friends or family members. One or more of the windows are *open* and you are sitting in the front seat. Can you understand the driver when his/her voice is loud enough for you and you can see his/her face?

52. You are the driver in an automobile with several friends or family members. The windows are *closed.* Can you understand the passenger behind you when his/her voice is loud enough for you?

53. You are the driver in an automobile with several friends or family members. One or more of the windows are *open.* Can you understand the passenger behind you when his/her voice is loud enough for you?

54. You are talking to a woman sitting in a ticket or information booth and it is fairly noisy. She is giving directions or information. Can you understand her when her voice is loud enough for you and you can see her face?

55. You are talking to a man sitting in a ticket or information booth and it is fairly noisy. He is giving directions or information. Can you understand him when his voice is loud enough for you and you can see his face?

56. You are in a room with background noise such as music or a crowd of people. Can you carry on a conversation with a person from another room if his/her voice is loud enough for you?

57. Can you hear an airplane in the sky when others around you can hear it?

58. Can you hear birds singing outside when others around you can hear them?

59. Can you hear water running in another room when others around you can hear it?

60. You are reading in a quiet room. Can you hear a person calling you from another room?

61. You are reading in a room with music or noise in the background. Can you hear a person calling you from another room?

62. You are at home reading in a quiet room. Do you hear the telephone ring when it is in another room?

63. You are at home watching television or listening to the radio. Can you hear the telephone ring when it is located in another room?

64. You are at home watching television or listening to the radio. Can you hear the doorbell ring when it is located in the *same* room?

65. You are at home watching television or listening to the radio. Can you hear the doorbell ring when it is located in *another* room?

66. When others are listening to speech on the television or radio, is it loud enough for you?

67. If you are riding in a car and you know that others are listening to music on the car radio, do you hear the music?

68. Do you find that children (6 to 10 years old) speak loudly enough for you?

69. When you are in your kitchen, do you hear the refrigerator motor going on and off?

70. You are in a quiet place and the person seated on the side of your better ear whispers to you. Can you hear the whisper?

71. How often do women speak loudly enough for you to hear them?

72. How often do men speak loudly enough for you to hear them?

73. When an announcement is given over a public-address system in a bus station or airport, is it loud enough for you to hear?

74. You are in a fairly quiet room and a person is talking to you from a distance of no more than six feet. Would you be aware that he/she is talking if you did not see his/her face?

75. A person is talking to you from a distance of no more than six feet. There is music or noise in the background. Would you be aware that he/she is talking if you did not see his/her face?

76. You are at a restaurant. When you miss something important that the waitress/ waiter said, do you ask for it to be repeated?

77. You are talking with a close friend. When you miss something important that was said, do you immediately adjust your hearing aid to help you hear better?

78. You are talking with five or six friends. When you miss something important that was said, do you ask the person talking to repeat it?

79. You are talking with a stranger. When you miss something important that was said, do you let him/her know that you have a hearing problem?

80. You are talking with a friend or family member. When you miss something important that was said, do you pretend you understood?

81. You are with a friend or family member and you hear only a portion of what was said. Do you repeat that portion before asking him/her for a repetition?

82. You are seated with five or six friends or family members around a table or in a living room. Often two persons are talking at once and one person frequently interrupts another. When you miss something important that was said, do you remind the person talking that you have a hearing problem?

83. You are talking with a friend or family member. When you miss something important that was said, do you ask for it to be repeated?

84. You are having dinner with five or six friends. When you miss something important that was said, do you let the person talking know you have a hearing problem?

85. At the beginning of a conversation, do you let a stranger know that you have a hearing problem?

86. You are seated with five or six strangers around a table or in a living room. Often two persons are talking at once and one person frequently interrupts another. When you miss something important that was said, do you pretend you understood?

87. You are seated with five or six strangers around a table or in a living room. Often two persons are talking at once and one person frequently interrupts another. When you miss something important that was said, do you let the person talking know you have a hearing problem?

88. You are with five or six friends or family members. One person at a time talks to the group. When you miss something important that was said, do you ask the person next to you?

89. You are seated with five or six friends around a table or in a living room. Often two persons are talking at once and one person frequently interrupts another.

When you miss something that was said, do you ask the person talking to repeat it?

90. You are at a restaurant and you hear only a portion of something the waitress/waiter said. Do you repeat the portion before asking him/her for a repetition?

91. You are with five or six strangers. One person at a time talks to the group. When you miss something important that was said, do you ask the person next to you?

92. You are with five or six strangers and you hear only a portion of what was said. Do you repeat that portion before asking the speaker for a repetition?

93. You are having dinner with five or six friends. When you miss something important that was said, do you ask the person talking to repeat it?

94. You are with five or six friends or family members. One person talks at a time. When you miss something important that was said, do you pretend you understood?

95. You are at a play, movie, or listening to a speech. When you miss something important that was said, do you ask the person with you?

96. You are talking with five or six strangers. When you miss something important that was said, do you ask the person talking to repeat it?

97. You are having dinner with five or six friends and you hear only a portion of what was said. Do you repeat that portion before asking the speaker for a repetition?

98. You are talking with a stranger. When you miss something important that was said, do you ask for it to be repeated?

99. You are with five or six friends or family members. One person at a time talks to the group. When you miss something important that was said, do you immediately adjust your hearing aid to help you hear better?

100. You are with five or six friends or family members and you hear only a portion of what was said. Do you repeat that portion before asking the speaker for a repetition?

101. You are talking with five or six strangers. When you miss something important that was said, do you let the person talking know you have a hearing problem?

102. You are at a small social gathering. If you have difficulty hearing what is being said, do you move to a place where you can hear better?

103. When you have difficulty understanding a person with a pipe, toothpick, or similar object in his/her mouth, do you ask him/her to remove the object?

104. When you are having difficulty following what someone is saying, do you keep trying until you are able to understand?

105. When you have difficulty understanding a person who speaks quite rapidly, do you ask him/her to speak more slowly?

106. You are at a committee meeting. If you have difficulty hearing what is being said, do you move to a place where you can hear better?

107. When you have difficulty understanding a person because he is holding his hand in front of his mouth, do you ask him to lower his hand?

108. You are at a lecture. If you have difficulty hearing what is being said, do you move to a place where you can hear better?

109. You are with a friend or family member in a fairly quiet room. Can you understand him/her when his/her voice is loud enough for you, but you can *not* see his/her face?

110. You are with a stranger in a fairly quiet room. Can you understand him/her when his/her voice is loud enough for you, but you can *not* see his/her face?

111. You are with a stranger and there is background noise such as music or a crowd of people. Can you understand the person when his/her voice is loud enough for you, but you can *not* see his/her face?

112. You are at a party or gathering of less than ten people and the room is fairly quiet. Can you understand what a friend or family member is saying to you when his/her voice is loud enough for you, but you can *not* see his/her face?

113. You are at a party or gathering of less than ten people and there is background noise such as music or a crowd of people. Can you understand what a friend or family member is saying to you when his/her voice is loud enough for you, but you can not see his/her face?

114. You are at a party or gathering of more than twenty people and there is background noise such as music or a crowd of people. Can you understand what a friend or family member is saying to you when his/her voice is loud enough for you, but you can *not* see his/her face?

115. You are at a party or gathering of more than twenty people and there is background noise such as music or a crowd of people. Can you understand what a stranger is saying to you when his/her voice is loud enough for you, but you can *not* see his/her face?

116. You are in a fairly quiet room with five or six friends or family members. One person talks at a time. When you are aware of the subject, can you understand what is being said when the speaker's voice is loud enough for you, but you can *not* see his/her face?

117. You are with five or six friends or family members and there is background noise such as music or a crowd of people. One person talks at a time. When you are aware of the subject, can you understand what is being said when the speakers voice is loud enough for you, but you can *not* see his/her face?

118. You are in a fairly quiet room with five or six strangers. One person talks at a time. When you are aware of the subject, you can understand what is being said when the speaker's voice is loud enough for you, but you can *not* see his/her face?

119. You are with five or six strangers and there is background noise such as music or a crowd of people. One person talks at a time. When you are aware of the subject, can you understand what is being said when the speaker's voice is loud enough for you, but you can *not* see his/her face?

120. You are in a fairly quiet room talking with five or six friends or family members. One person talks at a time. The subject of conversation changes from time to time. Can you understand what is being said when the speaker's voice is loud enough for you, but you can *not* see his/her face?

121. You are having dinner with five or six friends or family members at home and there is background noise such as music or a crowd of people. Can you understand what is being said when the speaker's voice is loud enough for you, but you can *not* see his/her face?

122. You are playing cards, monopoly, or some similar game and the room is fairly quiet. The subject of conversation changes from time to time. Can you understand what is being said when the speaker's voice is loud enough for you, but you can *not* see his/her face?

123. You are playing cards, monopoly, or some similar game and there is background noise such as music or a crowd of people. The subject of conversation changes from time to time. Can you understand what is being said when the speaker's voice is loud enough for you, but you can *not* see his/her face?

124. Does your hearing problem discourage you from going to the movies?

125. Does your hearing problem discourage you from attending lectures?

126. Does your hearing problem discourage you from going to concerts?

127. Does your hearing problem discourage you from going to plays?

128. Does your hearing problem lower your self-confidence?

129. Does your hearing problem tend to make you nervous and tense?

130. Does your hearing problem tend to make you impatient?

131. Do you feel that others cannot understand what it is to have a hearing problem?

## occupational items

132. You are with a female co-worker at work in a fairly quiet room. Can you understand her when her voice is loud enough for you and you can see her face?

133. You are with a male co-worker at work in a fairly quiet room. Can you understand him when his voice is loud enough for you and you can see his face?

134. You are with your employer (foreman, supervisor, etc.) at work in a fairly quiet room. Can you understand him when his voice is loud enough for you and you can see his face?

135. You are in a fairly quiet room at work with five or six co-workers. One person talks at a time. When you are aware of the subject, can you understand what is being said when the speaker's voice is loud enough for you and you can see his/her face?

136. You are in a fairly quiet room at work with five or six co-workers. One person talks at a time and the subject of conversation changes from time to time. Can you understand what is being said when the speaker's voice is loud enough for you and you can see his/her face?

137. You are with a female co-worker at work and several people are talking nearby. Can you understand her when her voice is loud enough for you and you can see her face?

138. You are with a female co-worker at work and there is background noise such as traffic, music, or a crowd of people. Can you understand her when her voice is loud enough for you and you can see her face?

139. You are with a male co-worker at work and several people are talking nearby. Can you understand him when his voice is loud enough for you and you can see his face?

140. You are with a male co-worker at work and there is background noise such as traffic, music, or a crowd of people. Can you understand him when his voice is loud enough for you and you can see his face?

141. You are with your employer (foreman, supervisor, etc.) and several people are talking nearby. Can you understand him/her when his/her voice is loud enough for you and you can see his/her face?

142. You are with your employer (foreman, supervisor, etc.) and there is background noise such as traffic, music, or a crowd of people. Can you understand him/her when his/her voice is loud enough for you and you can see his/her face?

143. You are at work with five or six co-workers and there is background noise such as music or a crowd of people. One person talks at a time and the subject of conversation changes from time to time. Can you understand what is being said when the speaker's voice is loud enough for you and you can see his/her face?

144. You are seated with five or six co-workers around a table at work. Often two persons are talking at once and one person frequently interrupts another. Can you understand what is being said when the speaker's voice is loud enough for you and you can see his/her face?

145. You are with five or six co-workers at work. One person talks at a time. When you miss something important that was said, do you pretend you understood?

146. You are talking with five or six co-workers at work. One person talks at a time. When you miss something important that was said, do you immediately adjust your hearing aid to help you hear better?

147. At the beginning of a conversation do you let your employer (foreman, supervisor, etc.) know that you have a hearing problem?

148. You are with a co-worker at work and you hear only a portion of what was said. Do you repeat that portion before asking the speaker for a repetition?

149. You are talking with your employer (foreman, supervisor, etc.) at work. When you miss something important that was said, do you pretend you understood?

150. At the beginning of a conversation, do you let your co-workers know that you have a hearing problem?

151. You are talking with a co-worker at work. When you miss something important that was said, do you immediately adjust your hearing aid to help you hear better?

152. You are talking with a co-worker at work. When you miss something important that was said, do you pretend you understood?

153. You are with your employer (foreman, supervisor, etc.) at work and you hear only a portion of what was said. Do you repeat that portion before asking the speaker for repetition?

154. You are talking with a co-worker or employer. When you miss something important that was said, do you let him/her know that you have a hearing problem?

155. You are talking with a co-worker at work. When you miss something important that was said, do you ask for it to be repeated?

156. Does your hearing problem interfere with helping or instructing others on the job?

157. Does your hearing problem interfere with your getting a job easily?

158. Does your hearing problem interfere with learning the duties of a new nob easily?

HEARING PERFORMANCE INVENTORY (EXPERIMENTAL FORM II)                    78-32P

NAME _____ AGE _____ DATE _____

ADDRESS _____ PHONE _____

TEST LOCATION _____ SEX _____ MARITAL STATUS_____

EMPLOYED _____ EDUCATION _____ HEARING AID WEARER: Yes ☐  No ☐

PRIOR AURAL REHABILITATION COURSE EXPERIENCE? _____ IF YES, WHEN? _____

This form can be obtained from the Speech Pathology Editor, Prentice-Hall, Inc., Englewood Cliffs, New Jersey 07632.

Index of items by numbers for HPI sections, categories, and subcategories. Within the categories and subcategories, the Social items are underlined and the Occupational items, are parenthesized. Formats follow tables in the text.

**sections**

*Understanding Speech:* 1–56; 109–123

    With Visual Cues: 1–7, 10–19, 23–51, 54–55
    With No Visual Cues: 8, 9, 20–22, 52–53, 56, 109–123

*Intensity:* 57–75

*Response to Auditory Failure:* 76–108

*Social:* 10–13, 35–53, 78, 82, 84, 86–89, 91–94, 96–97, 99–102, 106, 112–123

*Personal:* 124–131

*Occupational:* 132–158

    Understanding Speech: 132–144
    Response to Auditory Failure: 145–155
    Personal: 156–158

**categories and subcategories**

*Understanding Speech* (Visual Cues)

    *Talker (One-to-One): 1–7, 10–11, 14–15, 18–19, 25–42, 54–55, 132–134 137–142

      Male: 1, 4, 14, 18, 25, 28, 36, 39, 55 (133, 139, 140)
      Female: 2, 3, 15, 19, 26–27, 29, 37–38, 54 (132, 137, 138)
      Child: 5, 30, 31
      Friend/family member: 1, 2, 7, 10–11, 25–27, 34–35, 36–39, 41–42
      Stranger: 3, 4, 28, 29 40
      Co-worker: (132–133, 137–140)
      Employer: (134, 141–142)
      Waiter/waitress: 6, 32, 33

    Communicative Situation

      One-to-one (alone): 1–5, 7, 25–29, 30–31, 34–35, (132–134, 137–142)
      One-to-one in group < 10: 10, 36–37
      One-to-one in group > 20: 38–40
      One-to-one in group playing cards, etc.: 11, 41–42
      *Group conversation: 12–13, 43–48, 50–51 (135–136, 143–144)

        5 or 6 friends/family members: 12, 47
          Within group > 20: 43, 45–36

        5 or 6 strangers: 13, 48

          Within group > 20: 44

        5 or 6 co-workers: (135–136, 143–144)

Several friends in automobile: <u>50–51</u>
One talker at a time: <u>12</u>, <u>13</u>, <u>43–46</u> (135–136, 143)

Aware of subject: <u>12</u>, <u>43–44</u> (135)
Subject changes: <u>13</u>, <u>45–46</u> (136, 143)

Talkers interrupting: <u>48</u> (144)

Communication System

Public address (microphone) in auditorium: 18, 19
Television

News: 14, 15
Drama or movie: 16, 17

Movie: 23
Stage play: 24

Noise Environment

Fairly quiet: 1–7, <u>10–13</u>, 16, <u>50</u> (132–136)
Music, etc.: 17, 27–29, 31, 33, 35, <u>40</u>, <u>42–44</u>, <u>46–47</u>, <u>51</u>, 54–55 (138, 140)
People talking nearby: 25–26, 30, 32, 34, <u>36–39</u>, <u>41</u>, <u>45</u>, <u>49</u> (137, 139, 141)

Miscellaneous Situations

Restaurant: 6, 7, 32–35
Ticket or information booth: 54–55
Dinner: <u>47</u>

*Understanding Speech* (No Visual Cues):  8, 9, 20–22, 52–53, 56, 109–111, <u>112–123</u>

Talker (One-to-One)

Male: 8, 21
Female: 9, 22
Friend/family member: 109, <u>112–114</u>
Stranger: 110–111, <u>115</u>

Communicative Situation

One-to-one: 109–111
Other room: 8, 9, 56
One-to-one (group): <u>112–115</u>
*Group conversation: <u>52–53</u>, <u>116–123</u>

5 or 6 friends/family: <u>116–117</u>, <u>120–121</u>
5 or 6 strangers: <u>118–119</u>
Automobile: <u>52–53</u>
Games: <u>122–123</u>
One talker: <u>116–120</u>

Aware of subject: <u>116–119</u>
Subject changes: <u>120</u>, <u>122</u>, <u>123</u>

Communication System

Telephone: 21, 22
Public address in bus station: 20

Noise Environment

Fairly quiet: 8, 9, 52, 109–110, <u>112</u>, <u>116</u>, <u>118</u>, <u>120</u>, <u>122</u>
Music, etc.: <u>53</u>, 56, 111, <u>113–115</u>, <u>117</u>, <u>119</u>, <u>121</u>, <u>123</u>

*Intensity*

Talker

Male: 72
Female: 71
Child: 68

*Communicative Situation: 60–61, 70, 74–75

One-to-one: 70, 74, 75

Other room: 60–61
Six feet away: 74–75
Whisper: 70

Communication System

Public address in bus station or airport: 73
Radio or TV: 66, 67

Nonspeech

Doorbell

Same room: 64
Other room: 65

Telephone (other room): 62–63
Refrigerator: 69
Music (car radio): 67
Airplane: 57
Birds singing: 58
Water running: 59

Noise Environment

Quiet: 60, 62, 70, 74
Music, etc.: 61, 63–65, 75

*Response to Auditory Failure*

Talker (One-to-One)

Friend/family member: 77, 80–81, 83
Stranger: 79, 85, 98
Waiter/waitress: 76, 90
Co-worker: (148, 150–152, 154–155)
Employer: (147, 149, 153–154)

Communicative Situation

One-to-one: 76–77, 79–81, 83, 85, 90, 98 (147–155)
*Group conversation: 78, 82, 84, 86–89, 91–94, 96–97, 99–102 (145–146)

5 or 6 friends/family members: 78, 82, 84, 88–89, 93–94, 97, 99, 100
5 or 6 strangers: 86–87, 91–92, 96, 101
Small social gathering: 102
5 or 6 co-workers: (145–146)
One talker at a time: 88, 91, 94, 99 (145–146)
Talkers interrupting: 82, 86–87, 89

*Because items comprising the subheadings are not mutually exclusive, the items comprising the total category are provided.

Behavior Assessed

Adjust hearing aid: 77, <u>99</u> (146, 151)
Ask assistance or favor: <u>88</u>, <u>91</u>, 95, 103, 105, 107
Ask for repetition: 76, <u>78</u>, 83, <u>89</u>, <u>93</u>, <u>96</u>, 98 (155)
Ask for repeat of portion: 81, 90, <u>92</u>, <u>97</u>, <u>100</u> (148, 153)
Inform of hearing loss: 79, <u>82</u>, <u>84</u>, <u>85</u>, <u>87</u>, <u>101</u> (147, 150, 154)
Keep trying: 104
Move seat: <u>102</u>, <u>106</u>, 108
Pretend to understand: 80, <u>86</u>, <u>94</u> (145, 149, 152)

Miscellaneous Situations

Dinner: <u>84</u>, <u>93</u>, <u>97</u>
Restaurant: <u>76</u>, 90
Play, movie, lecture: 95, 108

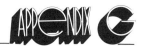

○ HEARING PERFORMANCE INVENTORY, REVISED FORM
Stanford H. Lamb, San Francisco State University; Elmer Owens, University of California; Earl D. Schubert, Stanford University; Thomas G. Giolas, University of Connecticut

**instructions**

We are interested in knowing how your hearing problem has affected your daily living. Below you will find a series of questions which describe a variety of everyday listening situations and ask you to judge how much difficulty you would have hearing in these situations.

Some of the questions ask you to judge how well you can understand what people are saying when their voices are loud enough. The term *understand* means hearing the words a person is saying clearly enough to be able to participate in the conversation. Other questions ask whether you can hear enough of a particular sound (doorbell, speech, etc.) to be aware of its presence. Other questions concern occupational, social, or personal situations. Still others ask what you *do* when you miss something. Always assume you are interested in what is being said.

To answer each question, you are asked to check the phrase that best describes how often you experience the situation being described:

Practically always . . . . . . . . . . . . . . . . . . . . . . . . . . . . . . . . .(or always)

Frequently . . . . . . . . . . . . . . . . . . .(about three-quarters of the time)

About half the time

Occasionally . . . . . . . . . . . . . . . . . . . . . . .(about a quarter of the time)

Almost never . . . . . . . . . . . . . . . . . . . . . . . . . . . . . . . . . . . .(or never)

For example, if you can understand what a person is saying on the telephone about 100% of the time, then you should check *practically always.* On the other hand, if you can understand almost nothing of what a person is saying on the telephone, then you should check *almost never.* If you can understand what a person is saying on the telephone about 50% of the time, then you should check *about half the time.*

Your answers to the questions should describe your present hearing ability as it is on the average rather than from a single instance.

If you wear a hearing aid in the situation described, answer the question accordingly.

Please check *one, and only one,* phrase for each question. You should check *does not apply* only if you have not experienced a particular situation or one similar to it.

Questions that appear identical do differ in at least one important detail. Please read each question carefully before checking the appropriate phrase.

We know that people talk differently. Some mumble, others talk too fast, and others talk without moving their lips very much. Please answer the questions according to the way *most* people talk to you.

If the question does not specify whether the person speaking is male or female, answer according to which sex you have the most difficulty hearing.

Asterisks on the score sheet are for scoring purposes and should be ignored.

1. You are watching your favorite news program on television. Can you understand the news reporter (female) when her voice is loud enough for you?

2. You are reading in a room with music or noise in the background. Can you hear a person calling you from another room?

3. You are with a male friend or family member in a fairly quiet room. Can you understand him when his voice is loud enough for you and you can see his face?

4. Can you hear an airplane in the sky when others around you can hear it?

5. You are watching a drama or movie on television. Can you understand what is being said when the speaker's voice is loud enough for you and there is music in the background?

6. Can you understand what a woman is saying on the telephone when her voice is loud enough for you?

7. You are at a restaurant and you hear only a portion of something the waitress/waiter said. Do you repeat the portion when asking him/her for a repetition?

8. You are with a child (6 to 10 years old) in a fairly quiet room. Can you understand the child when his/her voice is loud enough for you and you can see his/her face?

9. You are the driver in an automobile with several friends or family members. One or more of the windows are open. Can you understand the passenger behind you when his/her voice is loud enough for you?

10. You are at a restaurant and there is background noise such as music or a crowd of people. Can you understand the waiter/waitress when his/her voice is loud enough for you and you can see his/her face?

11. You are talking with a close friend. When you miss something important that was said, do you immediately adjust your hearing aid to help you hear better?

12. You are with five or six strangers at a gathering of more than twenty people and there is background noise such as music or a crowd of people. One person talks at a time. When you are aware of the subject, can you understand

what is being said when the speaker's voice is loud enough for you and you can see his/her face?

13. You are at a play or movie or listening to a speech. When you miss something important that was said, do you ask the person with you?

14. You are with a child (6 to 10 years old) and several people are talking nearby. Can you understand the child when his/her voice is loud enough for you and you can see his/her face?

15. You are playing cards, monopoly, or some similar game with several people and there is background noise such as music or a crowd of people. Can you understand what a friend or family member is saying to you when his/her voice is loud enough for you and you can see his/her face?

16. Does your hearing problem discourage you from attending lectures?

17. You are talking with five or six friends. When you miss something that was said, do you ask the person talking to repeat it?

18. You are in an auditorium listening to a lecturer (female) who is using a microphone. Can you understand what she is saying when her voice is loud enough for you and you can see her face?

19. Can you hear water running in another room when others around you can hear it?

20. You are with a friend or family member and you hear only a portion of what was said. Do you repeat that portion when asking him/her for a repetition?

21. You are at a party or gathering of less than ten people and the room is fairly quiet. Can you understand what a friend or family member is saying to you when his/her voice is loud enough for you but you can *not* see his/her face?

22. Does your hearing problem lower your self-confidence?

23. You are in a fairly quiet room with five or six strangers. One person talks at a time. When you are aware of the subject, can you understand what is being said when the speaker's voice is loud enough for you but you can *not* see his/her face?

24. You are with five or six friends or family members at a gathering of more than twenty people and several people are talking nearby. One person talks at a time and the subject of conversation changes from time to time. Can you understand what is being said when the speaker's voice is loud enough for you and you can see his/her face?

25. When an announcement is given over a public-address system in a bus station or airport, is it *loud enough* for you to hear?

26. You are talking with a stranger. When you miss something important that was said, do you ask for it to be repeated?

27. You are talking with a friend or family member. When you miss something that was said, do you pretend you understood?

28. You are at a fairly quiet restaurant. Can you understand the waiter/waitress when his/her voice is loud enough for you and you can see his/her face?

29. You are seated with five or six strangers around a table or in a living room. Often two persons are talking at once and one person frequently interrupts another. When you miss something important that was said, do you pretend you understood?

30. You are playing cards, monopoly, or some similar game and the room is fairly quiet. The subject of conversation changes from time to time. Can you understand what is being said when the speaker's voice is loud enough for you but you can *not* see his/her face?

31. You are at a party or gathering of less than ten people and the room is fairly quiet. Can you understand what a friend or family member is saying to you when his/her voice is loud enough for you and you can see his/her face?

32. Does your hearing problem discourage you from going to concerts?

33. Do you find that children (6 to 10 years old) speak loudly enough for you?

34. When an announcement is given over a public-address system in a bus station or airport, can you understand what is being said when the speaker's voice is loud enough for you?

35. You are seated with five or six strangers around a table or in a living room. Often two persons are talking at once and one person frequently interrupts another. Can you understand what is being said when the speaker's voice is loud enough for you and you can see his/her face?

36. You are seated with five or six friends around a table or in a living room. Often two persons are talking at once and one person frequently interrupts another. When you miss something that was said, do you ask the person talking to repeat it?

37. You are with a female stranger in a fairly quiet room. Can you understand her when her voice is loud enough for you and you can see her face?

38. You are with a stranger and there is background noise such as music or a crowd of people. Can you understand the person when his/her voice is loud enough for you but you can *not* see his/her face?

39. Does your hearing problem tend to make you impatient?

40. You are talking with five or six strangers. When you miss something important that was said, do you let the person talking know, at least one time, that you have a hearing problem?

41. You are at a party or gathering of less than ten people and several people are talking nearby. Can you understand what a friend or family member (female) is saying to you when her voice is loud enough for you and you can see her face?

42. Does your hearing problem discourage you from going to plays?

43. You are having dinner with five or six friends and you hear only a portion of what was said. Do you repeat that portion when asking the speaker for a repetition?

44. You are at a restaurant with a friend or family member and there is background noise such as music or a crowd of people. Can you understand the person when his/her voice is loud enough for you and you can see his/her face?

45. When you have difficulty understanding a person who speaks quite rapidly, do you ask him/her to speak more slowly?

46. You are talking to a woman sitting in a ticket or information booth and it is fairly noisy. She is giving directions or information. Can you understand her when her voice is loud enough for you and you can see her face?

47. You are having dinner with five or six friends. When you miss something important that was said, do you ask the person talking to repeat it?

48. When others are listening to speech on the television or radio, is it loud enough for you?

49. Does your hearing problem discourage you from going to the movies?

50. You are riding in an automobile with several friends or family members. One or more of the windows are open and you are sitting in the front seat. Can you understand the driver when his/her voice is loud enough for you and you can see his/her face?

51. You are at home watching television or listening to the radio. Can you hear the doorbell ring when it is located in the same room?

52. You are in a fairly quiet room talking with five or six strangers. One person talks at a time and the subject of conversation changes from time to time. Can you understand what is being said when the speaker's voice is loud enough for you and you can see his/her face?

53. You are seated with five or six friends or family members around a table or in a living room. Often two persons are talking at once and one person frequently interrupts another. When you miss something important that was said, do you remind the person talking, at least once, that you have a hearing problem?

54. You are attending a stage play. Can you understand what the actors/actresses are saying when their voices are loud enough for you and you can see their faces?

55. You are with a friend or family member in a fairly quiet room. Can you understand him/her when his/her voice is loud enough for you but you can *not* see his/her face?

56. A person is talking to you from a distance of no more than six feet. There is music or noise in the background. Would you be aware that he/she is talking if you did not see his/her face?

57. You are having dinner with five or six friends or family members at home and there is background noise such as music or a crowd of people. Can you understand what is being said when the speaker's voice is loud enough for you but you can *not* see his/her face?

58. When you have difficulty understanding a person with a pipe, toothpick, or similar object in his/her mouth, do you ask him/her to remove the object?

59. You are the driver in an automobile with several friends or family members. The windows are closed. Can you understand the passenger behind you when his/her voice is loud enough for you?

60. When you have difficulty understanding a person because he is holding his hand in front of his mouth, do you ask him to lower his hand?

61. You are at a party or gathering of more than twenty people and there is background noise such as music or a crowd of people. Can you understand what a stranger is saying to you when his/her voice is loud enough for you and you can see his/her face?

62. Do you feel that others cannot understand what it is to have a hearing problem?

63. You are at a movie. Can you understand what the actors/actresses are saying when their voices are loud enough for you and you can see their faces?

64. You are talking with five or six strangers. When you miss something important that was said, do you ask the person talking to repeat it?

65. You are at a party or gathering of more than twenty people and several people are talking nearby. Can you understand what a friend or family member (male) is saying to you when his voice is loud enough for you and you can see his face?

66. You are in a fairly quiet room. Can you carry on a conversation with a man in another room if his voice is loud enough for you?

67. You are with a male friend or family member and several people are talking nearby. Can you understand him when his voice is loud enough for you and you can see his face?

68. You are with five or six friends or family members. One person talks at a time. When you miss something important that was said, do you pretend you understood?

69. You are watching a drama or movie on television. Can you understand what is being said when the speaker's voice is loud enough for you and there is no music in the background?

70. You are with five or six friends or family members and there is background noise such as music or a crowd of people. One person talks at a time. When you are aware of the subject, can you understand what is being said when the speaker's voice is loud enough for you but you can *not* see his/her face?

71. You are at a lecture. If you have difficulty hearing what is being said, do you move to a place where you can hear better?

72. Does your hearing problem tend to make you feel nervous or tense?

73. You are with a female stranger and there is background noise such as traffic, music, or a crowd of people. Can you understand her when her voice is loud enough for you and you can see her face?

74. You are in a quiet place and the person seated on the side of your better ear whispers to you. Can you hear the whisper?

75. You are at a small social gathering. If you have difficulty hearing what is being said, do you move to a place where you can hear better?

### occupational items

76. You are with a male co-worker at work in a fairly quiet room. Can you understand him when his voice is loud enough for you and you can see his face?

77. You are with five or six co-workers at work. One person talks at a time. When you miss something important that was said, do you pretend you understand?

78. Does your hearing problem interfere with helping or instructing others on the job?

79. You are with a female co-worker at work and there is background noise such as traffic, music, or a crowd of people. Can you understand her when her voice is loud enough for you and you can see her face?

80. You are with a co-worker at work and you hear only a portion of what was said. Do you repeat that portion when asking the speaker for a repetition?

81. You are talking with a co-worker at work. When you miss something important that was said, do you ask for it to be repeated?

82. You are talking with your employer (foreman, supervisor, etc.) and several people are talking nearby. Can you understand him/her when his/her voice is loud enough for you and you can see his/her face?

83. You are with a female co-worker at work in a fairly quiet room. Can you understand her when her voice is loud enough for you and you can see her face?

84. You are talking with a co-worker or employer. When you miss something important that was said, do you remind him/her that you have a hearing problem?

85. You are in a fairly quiet room at work with five or six co-workers. One person talks at a time and the subject of conversation changes from time to time. Can you understand what is being said when the speaker's voice is loud enough for you and you can see his/her face?

86. Does your hearing problem interfere with learning the duties of a new job easily?

87. You are seated with five or six co-workers around a table at work. Often two persons are talking at once and one person frequently interrupts another. Can you understand what is being said when the speaker's voice is loud enough for you and you can see his/her face?

88. You are talking with a co-worker at work. When you miss something important that was said, do you pretend you understood?

89. You are with a male co-worker at work and there is background noise such as traffic, music, or a crowd of people. Can you understand him when his voice is loud enough for you and you can see his face?

90. You are talking with a co-worker at work. When you miss something that was said, do you immediately adjust your hearing aid to help you hear better?

## sections

*Understanding Speech*
    With Visual Cues 1, 3, 5, 8, 10, 12, 14, 15, 18, 24, 28, 31, 35, 37, 41, 44 46, 50, 52, 54, 61, 63, 65, 67, 69, 73
    With No Visual Cues 6, 9, 21, 23, 30, 34, 38, 55, 57, 59, 66, 70

*Intensity* 2, 4, 19, 25, 33, 48, 51, 56, 74

*Response to Auditory Failure* 7, 11, 13, 17, 20, 26, 27, 29, 36, 40, 43, 47, 53, 58, 60, 64, 68, 71, 75

*Personal* 16, 22, 32, 39, 42, 49, 62, 72

*Social* 9, 12, 15, 17, 21, 23, 24, 29, 30, 31, 35, 36, 40, 41, 43, 47, 50, 52, 53, 57, 59, 61, 64, 65, 68, 70, 75

79-334P

HEARING PERFORMANCE INVENTORY (REVISED FORM)

NAME ______ AGE ______ DATE ______

ADDRESS ______ PHONE ______

TEST LOCATION ______ SEX ______ MARITAL STATUS ______

EMPLOYED ______ EDUCATION ______ HEARING AID WEARER: Yes ☐ No ☐

PRIOR AURAL REHABILITATION COURSE EXPERIENCE? ______ IF YES, WHEN? ______

| | Practically Always | Frequently | About Half The Time | Occasionally | Almost Never | Does Not Apply | | Practically Always | Frequently | About Half The Time | Occasionally | Almost Never | Does Not Apply |
|---|---|---|---|---|---|---|---|---|---|---|---|---|---|
| 1. | ☐ | ☐ | ☐ | ☐ | ☐ — | ☐ | 46. | ☐ | ☐ | ☐ | ☐ | ☐ — | ☐ |
| 2. | ☐ | ☐ | ☐ | ☐ | ☐ — | ☐ | 47. | ☐ | ☐ | ☐ | ☐ | ☐ — | ☐ |
| 3. | ☐ | ☐ | ☐ | ☐ | ☐ — | ☐ | 48. | ☐ | ☐ | ☐ | ☐ | ☐ — | ☐ |
| 4. | ☐ | ☐ | ☐ | ☐ | ☐ — | ☐ | * 49. | ☐ | ☐ | ☐ | ☐ | ☐ — | ☐ |
| 5. | ☐ | ☐ | ☐ | ☐ | ☐ — | ☐ | 50. | ☐ | ☐ | ☐ | ☐ | ☐ — | ☐ |
| 6. | ☐ | ☐ | ☐ | ☐ | ☐ — | ☐ | 51. | ☐ | ☐ | ☐ | ☐ | ☐ — | ☐ |
| 7. | ☐ | ☐ | ☐ | ☐ | ☐ — | ☐ | 52. | ☐ | ☐ | ☐ | ☐ | ☐ — | ☐ |
| 8. | ☐ | ☐ | ☐ | ☐ | ☐ — | ☐ | 53. | ☐ | ☐ | ☐ | ☐ | ☐ — | ☐ |
| 9. | ☐ | ☐ | ☐ | ☐ | ☐ — | ☐ | 54. | ☐ | ☐ | ☐ | ☐ | ☐ — | ☐ |
| 10. | ☐ | ☐ | ☐ | ☐ | ☐ — | ☐ | 55. | ☐ | ☐ | ☐ | ☐ | ☐ — | ☐ |
| 11. | ☐ | ☐ | ☐ | ☐ | ☐ — | ☐ | 56. | ☐ | ☐ | ☐ | ☐ | ☐ — | ☐ |
| 12. | ☐ | ☐ | ☐ | ☐ | ☐ — | ☐ | 57. | ☐ | ☐ | ☐ | ☐ | ☐ — | ☐ |
| 13. | ☐ | ☐ | ☐ | ☐ | ☐ — | ☐ | 58. | ☐ | ☐ | ☐ | ☐ | ☐ — | ☐ |
| 14. | ☐ | ☐ | ☐ | ☐ | ☐ — | ☐ | 59. | ☐ | ☐ | ☐ | ☐ | ☐ — | ☐ |
| 15. | ☐ | ☐ | ☐ | ☐ | ☐ — | ☐ | 60. | ☐ | ☐ | ☐ | ☐ | ☐ — | ☐ |
| * 16. | ☐ | ☐ | ☐ | ☐ | ☐ — | ☐ | 61. | ☐ | ☐ | ☐ | ☐ | ☐ — | ☐ |
| 17. | ☐ | ☐ | ☐ | ☐ | ☐ — | ☐ | * 62. | ☐ | ☐ | ☐ | ☐ | ☐ — | ☐ |
| 18. | ☐ | ☐ | ☐ | ☐ | ☐ — | ☐ | 63. | ☐ | ☐ | ☐ | ☐ | ☐ — | ☐ |
| 19. | ☐ | ☐ | ☐ | ☐ | ☐ — | ☐ | 64. | ☐ | ☐ | ☐ | ☐ | ☐ — | ☐ |
| 20. | ☐ | ☐ | ☐ | ☐ | ☐ — | ☐ | 65. | ☐ | ☐ | ☐ | ☐ | ☐ — | ☐ |
| 21. | ☐ | ☐ | ☐ | ☐ | ☐ — | ☐ | 66. | ☐ | ☐ | ☐ | ☐ | ☐ — | ☐ |
| * 22. | ☐ | ☐ | ☐ | ☐ | ☐ — | ☐ | 67. | ☐ | ☐ | ☐ | ☐ | ☐ — | ☐ |
| 23. | ☐ | ☐ | ☐ | ☐ | ☐ — | ☐ | * 68. | ☐ | ☐ | ☐ | ☐ | ☐ — | ☐ |
| 24. | ☐ | ☐ | ☐ | ☐ | ☐ — | ☐ | 69. | ☐ | ☐ | ☐ | ☐ | ☐ — | ☐ |
| 25. | ☐ | ☐ | ☐ | ☐ | ☐ — | ☐ | 70. | ☐ | ☐ | ☐ | ☐ | ☐ — | ☐ |
| 26. | ☐ | ☐ | ☐ | ☐ | ☐ — | ☐ | 71. | ☐ | ☐ | ☐ | ☐ | ☐ — | ☐ |
| * 27. | ☐ | ☐ | ☐ | ☐ | ☐ — | ☐ | * 72. | ☐ | ☐ | ☐ | ☐ | ☐ — | ☐ |
| 28. | ☐ | ☐ | ☐ | ☐ | ☐ — | ☐ | 73. | ☐ | ☐ | ☐ | ☐ | ☐ — | ☐ |
| * 29. | ☐ | ☐ | ☐ | ☐ | ☐ — | ☐ | 74. | ☐ | ☐ | ☐ | ☐ | ☐ — | ☐ |
| 30. | ☐ | ☐ | ☐ | ☐ | ☐ — | ☐ | 75. | ☐ | ☐ | ☐ | ☐ | ☐ — | ☐ |
| 31. | ☐ | ☐ | ☐ | ☐ | ☐ — | ☐ | 76. | ☐ | ☐ | ☐ | ☐ | ☐ — | ☐ |
| * 32. | ☐ | ☐ | ☐ | ☐ | ☐ — | ☐ | * 77. | ☐ | ☐ | ☐ | ☐ | ☐ — | ☐ |
| 33. | ☐ | ☐ | ☐ | ☐ | ☐ — | ☐ | * 78. | ☐ | ☐ | ☐ | ☐ | ☐ — | ☐ |
| 34. | ☐ | ☐ | ☐ | ☐ | ☐ — | ☐ | 79. | ☐ | ☐ | ☐ | ☐ | ☐ — | ☐ |
| 35. | ☐ | ☐ | ☐ | ☐ | ☐ — | ☐ | 80. | ☐ | ☐ | ☐ | ☐ | ☐ — | ☐ |
| 36. | ☐ | ☐ | ☐ | ☐ | ☐ — | ☐ | 81. | ☐ | ☐ | ☐ | ☐ | ☐ — | ☐ |
| 37. | ☐ | ☐ | ☐ | ☐ | ☐ — | ☐ | 82. | ☐ | ☐ | ☐ | ☐ | ☐ — | ☐ |
| 38. | ☐ | ☐ | ☐ | ☐ | ☐ — | ☐ | 83. | ☐ | ☐ | ☐ | ☐ | ☐ — | ☐ |
| * 39. | ☐ | ☐ | ☐ | ☐ | ☐ — | ☐ | 84. | ☐ | ☐ | ☐ | ☐ | ☐ — | ☐ |
| 40. | ☐ | ☐ | ☐ | ☐ | ☐ — | ☐ | 85. | ☐ | ☐ | ☐ | ☐ | ☐ — | ☐ |
| 41. | ☐ | ☐ | ☐ | ☐ | ☐ — | ☐ | * 86. | ☐ | ☐ | ☐ | ☐ | ☐ — | ☐ |
| * 42. | ☐ | ☐ | ☐ | ☐ | ☐ — | ☐ | 87. | ☐ | ☐ | ☐ | ☐ | ☐ — | ☐ |
| 43. | ☐ | ☐ | ☐ | ☐ | ☐ — | ☐ | * 88. | ☐ | ☐ | ☐ | ☐ | ☐ — | ☐ |
| 44. | ☐ | ☐ | ☐ | ☐ | ☐ — | ☐ | 89. | ☐ | ☐ | ☐ | ☐ | ☐ — | ☐ |
| 45. | ☐ | ☐ | ☐ | ☐ | ☐ — | ☐ | 90. | ☐ | ☐ | ☐ | ☐ | ☐ — | ☐ |

* Items to be reversed before scoring.

This form can be obtained from the Speech Pathology Editor, Prentice-Hall, Inc., Englewood Cliffs, New Jersey 07632.

*Occupational*

Understanding Speech with Visual Cues 76, 79, 82, 83, 85, 87, 89
Response to Auditory Failure 77, 80, 81, 84, 88, 90
Personal 78, 86

**categories and subcategories**

Social items are underlined, occupational items parenthesized.

*Understanding Speech (with Visual Cues)*

Talker
  Male 3, 67, 65 (76, 89)
  Female 37, 1, 18, 73, 41, 46 (83, 79)
  Child 8, 14
  Friend/family member 3, 31, 67, 44, 41, 65, 15
  Stranger 37, 73, 61
  Co-worker (83, 76, 79, 89)
  Employer (82)
  Waiter/waitress 28, 10

Communicative Situation

  One-to-one 3, 37, 8, 31, 67, 73, 14, 44, 41, 65, 61, 15 (83, 76, 79, 89, 82)
    Alone 3, 37, 8, 67, 73, 14, 44 (83, 76, 79, 89, 82)
    In group<10 31, 41
    In group>20 65, 61,
    In group playing cards, etc. 15
  Group conversation 52, 12, 24, 35, 50 (85, 87)
    5 or 6 friends/family members within group>20 24
    5 or 6 strangers 52, 35
      Within group>20 12
    5 or 6 co-workers (85, 87)
    Several friends in automobile 50
    One talker at a time
      Listener aware of subject 12
      Subject changes 52, 24 (85)
    Talkers interrupting 35 (87)

Communication System
  Public address in auditorium 18
  Television
    News 1
    Drama or Movie 69, 5
  Movie 63
  Stage play 54

Noise Environment
  Fairly quiet 3, 37, 8, 28, 31, 52, 69 (83, 76, 85)
  Music, etc. 5, 73, 10, 44, 61, 15, 12, 50, 46 (79, 89)
  People talking nearby 67, 14, 41, 65, 24 (82)

Miscellaneous
  Restaurant 28, 10, 44
  Ticket or information booth 46

*Understanding Speech (No Visual Cues)*

Talker
  Male 66
  Female 6

Friend/family member 55, <u>21</u>
Stranger, 38
Communicative Situation
One-to-one 66, 55, 38, 21
Alone 55, 38
Other room 66
In group <u>21</u>
Group conversation, <u>59</u>, <u>9</u>, <u>70</u>, <u>23</u>, <u>57</u>, <u>30</u>
5 or 6 friends/family members <u>70</u>, <u>57</u>
5 or 6 strangers <u>23</u>
Automobile <u>59</u>, <u>9</u>
Games <u>30</u>
One talker at a time
Listener aware of subject <u>70</u>, 23
Subject changes <u>30</u>
Comminication System
Telephone 6
Public address in bus station 34
Noise Environment
Fairly quiet 66, <u>59</u>, <u>55</u>, <u>21</u>, <u>23</u>, <u>30</u>
Music, etc. <u>9</u>, 38, <u>70</u>, <u>57</u>

*Intensity*

Talker
Child 33
Communicative Situation (One-to-One)
Other room 2
Six feet away 56
Whisper 74
Communication System
Public address in bus station or airport 25
Radio or TV 48
Nonspeech
Doorbell (same room) 51
Airplane 4
Water running 19

Noise Environment
Quiet 74
Music, etc. 2, 51, 56

*Response to Auditory Failure*

Talker
Friend/family member 11, 27, 20
Stranger 26
Waiter/waitress 7
Co-worker (80, 90, 88, 84, 81)
Employer (84)

Communicative Situation

One-to-one 11, 27, 20, 7, 26 (80, 90, 88, 84, 81)
Group conversation 17, 53, 29, 36, 47, 68, 64, 43, 40, 75 (77)
    5 or 6 friends/family members 17, 53, 36, 47, 68, 42
    5 or 6 strangers 29, 64, 40
    Small social gathering 75
    5 or 6 co-workers 77
    One talker at a time 68 (77)
    Talkers interrupting 53, 29, 36

Behavior Assessed

Adjust hearing aid 11, (1, 3)
Ask assistance or favor 13, 58, 45, 60
Ask for repetition 17, 36, 47, 64, 26 (81)
Ask for repeat of portion 20, 7, 43 (80)
Inform of hearing loss 53, 40 (84)
Move seat 75, 71
Pretend to understand 27, 29, 68 (77, 88)

Miscellaneous

Dinner 47, 43
Restaurant 7
Play, movie, Lecture 13, 71

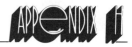

○ THE DENVER SCALE OF COMMUNICATION FUNCTION
FOR SENIOR CITIZENS LIVING IN RETIREMENT
CENTERS*

NAME_____DATE OF PRE-TEST_____
ADDRESS_____DATE OF POST-TEST_____
AGE_____EXAMINER _____
SEX_____

1. Do you have trouble communicating with your family because of your hearing
   problem? Yes__ No__
   Probe Effect I:
   a. Does your family make decisions for you because of your hearing problem?
      Yes__ No__
   b. Does your family leave you out of discussions because of your hearing
      problem? Yes__ No__
   c. Does your family get angry or annoyed with you because of your hearing
      problem? Yes__ No__
   Exploration Effect:
   a. Do you have a family? Yes__ No__
   b. How often does your family visit you?_____
   c. How far away does your family live? In a city____ Other____
   d. How often do you visit your family?_____

2. Do you get upset when you cannot hear or understand what is being
   said? Yes__ No__
   Probe Effect I (to be used only if person responds yes):
   a. Do your friends know you get upset? Yes__ No__
   b. Does your family know you get upset? Yes__ No__
   c. Does the staff know you get upset? Yes__ No__
   Probe Effect II (to be used only if person responds no):
   a. Do your friends realize you are not upset? Yes__ No__

*Janet M. Zarnoch and Jerome G. Alpiner, unpublished study. The University of
Denver, © 1976. Reprinted by permission.

b. Does your family realize you are not upset? Yes__ No__

c. Does the staff realize you are not upset? Yes__ No__

Exploration Effect (to be used only if person responds yes):

a. How does your behavior change when you become upset?

3. Do you think your family, your friends, and the staff understand what it is like to have a hearing problem? Yes__ No__

Probe Effect:

a. Do they avoid you because of your hearing problem? Yes__ No__

b. Do they leave you out of discussions? Yes__ No__

c. Do they hesitate to ask you to socialize with them? Yes__ No__

Exploration Effect:

a. Family Yes__ No__

b. Friends Yes__ No__

c. Staff Yes__ No__

4. Do you avoid communicating with other people because of your hearing problem? Yes__ No__

Probe Effect:

a. Do you communicate with people during meal times? Yes__ No__

b. Do you communicate with your roommate(s)? Yes__ No__

c. Do you communicate during the social activities in the home? Yes__ No__

d. Do you communicate with visiting family or friends? Yes__ No__

e. Do you communicate with the staff? Yes__ No__

Exploration Effect:

a. Is your roommate capable of communication? Yes__ No__

b. What are the social activities of the home? _____

c. Which ones do you attend? _____

5. Do you feel that you are a relaxed person? Yes__ No__

Probe Effect:

a. Do you think you are an irritable person because of your hearing problem? Yes__ No__

b. Do you think you are an irritable person because of your age? Yes__ No__

c. Do you think you are an irritable person because you live in this home? Yes__ No__

Exploration Effect:

a. Do you have to live in this home? Yes__ No__

6. Do you feel relaxed in group communicative situations? Yes__ No__

Probe Effect:

a. Do you get nervous when you have to ask people to repeat what they have said if you have not understood them? Yes__ No__

  b. Do you feel nervous if you have to tell a person that you have a hearing problem? Yes__ No__

Exploration Effect:

  a. Do you watch facial expressions? Yes__ No__

  b. Do you watch gestures? Yes__ No__

  c. Do you think you are a good listener? Yes__ No__ Why?

  d. Do you have a hearing aid? Yes__ No__

  e. Do you wear your aid? Yes__ No__

---

7. Do you think you need help in overcoming your hearing problem? Yes__ No__

Probe Effect:

  a. If lipreading training was available, would you attend? Yes__ No__

  b. Do you think this home provides adequate activities to make you want to communicate? Yes__ No__

Exploration Effect I:

  a. Can a person improve his communication ability by using lipreading (or speechreading), which means watching the speaker's lips, facial expressions, and gestures when he's speaking to you? Yes__ No__

  b. Do you agree with the above as a definition of lipreading? Yes__ No__

Exploration Effect II:

  a. Is your vision adequate? Yes__ No__

  b. Are you able to get around unassisted? Yes__ No__

NAME_____  DATE OF PRETEST_____
ADDRESS_____  DATE OF POSTTEST_____
AGE_____  EXAMINER_____  SEX_____

| CATEGORY | MAIN QUESTION | PROBE EFFECTS | EXPLORATION EFFECTS | PROBLEM | NO PROBLEM |
|---|---|---|---|---|---|
| Family | 1. + [ ] − [ ] | a [ ] b [ ] c [ ] | a. ___ b. ___ c. ___ d. ___ | | |
| Emotional | 2. [ ] [ ] | I a [ ] b [ ] c [ ]  II a [ ] b [ ] c [ ] | a. ___ | | |
| Other Persons | 3. [ ] [ ] | a [ ] b [ ] c [ ] | a. ___ b. ___ c. ___ | | |
| General Communication | 4. [ ] [ ] | a [ ] b [ ] c [ ] d [ ]  e [ ] | a. ___ b. ___ c. ___ | | |

| CATEGORY | MAIN QUESTION | PROBE EFFECTS | EXPLORATION EFFECTS | PROBLEM | NO PROBLEM |
|---|---|---|---|---|---|
| Self Concept | 5. ☐ ☐ | a ☐  b ☐  c ☐ | a. _____ | | |
| Group Situations | 6. ☐ ☐ | a ☐  b ☐ | a. _____ <br> b. _____ <br> c. _____ <br> d. _____ <br> e. _____ | | |
| Rehabilitation | 7. ☐ ☐ | a ☐  b ☐ | Ia. _____ <br> b. _____ <br> IIa. _____ <br> b. _____ | | |

Key + = person responded yes to question
      − = person responded no to question

Additional Client Comments: 1. _____

2. _____

3. _____

4. _____

5. _____

6. _____

7. _____

Examiner _____ Date _____

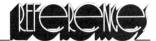

ALPINER, J. G. ed. "Evaluation of Communication Function," in *Handbook of Rehabilitative Audiology*, Baltimore: Williams and Wilkins, 1978, pp. 30–66.

ALPINER, J. G. ed., "Rehabilitation of the Geriatric Client," in *Handbook of Rehabilitative Audiology*, Baltimore: Williams and Wilkins, 1978, pp. 141–172.

ALPINER, J. G. "Psychological and Social Aspects of Aging as Related to Hearing Rehabilitation of Elderly Clients," in *Aural Rehabilitation for the Elderly*, M. Henoch ed., New York: Grune and Stratton, Inc., 1979, pp. 169–184.

ALPINER, J. G, W. CHEVRETTE, G. GLASCOE, M. METZ, and B. OLSEN, "The Denver Scale of Communication Function," unpublished study, Denver, Colorado: University of Denver, 1971.

AMERICAN NATIONAL STANDARDS SPECIFICATIONS FOR AUDIOMETERS, 1969. S3.6, American National Standards Institute, New York.

AMERICAN SPEECH and HEARING ASSOCIATION COMMITTEE ON REHABILITATIVE AUDIOLOGY, "The Audiologist's Responsibilities,' *ASHA*, 16(1974), pp. 68–70.

AMERICAN SPEECH and HEARING ASSOCIATION TASK FORCE, Definition of Hearing Handicap, 1980.

AMERICAN STANDARDS ASSOCIATION SPECIFICATIONS FOR SPEECH AUDIOMETERS, ASA, Z24.13-1953. New York: U.S.A. Standards Institute, 1953.

ARGYLE, M. *The Psychology of Interpersonal Behavior.* New York: Penquin Books, 1978.

ATHERLEY, G. and W. NOBLE, "Clinical Picture of Occupational Hearing Loss Obtained with the Hearing Measurement Scale," in *Occupational Hearing Loss,* D. W. Robinson ed., London, England: Academic Press, 1971, pp. 193–206.

BARKER, L. D., J. CEGALA, R. J. KIBLER, and K. J. WAHLERS, *Groups in Process: An Introduction to Small Group Communication.* Englewood Cliffs, New Jersey: Prentice-Hall, Inc., 1979.

BERGER, K. A. "Speech Discrimination Task Using Multiple Choice Key Words in Sentences," *Journal of Auditory Research,* 12(1969), pp. 247–262.

BERKOWITZ, A. O. and I. HOCHBERG, "Self-Assessment of Hearing Handicap in the Aged," *Archives of Otolaryngology,* 93(1971), pp. 25–28.

BEVAN, M. A. "The Effectiveness of the Hearing Performance Inventory with a Hearing-Impaired Population—A Pilot Study," unpublished manuscript, Storrs, Connecticut: University of Connecticut, Department of Speech, 1977.

BERGMAN, M., V. BLUMENFELD, D. CASCARDO, B. DASH, H. LEVITT, and M. MARGULIES, "Age-Related Decrement in Hearing for Speech, *Journal of Gerontology,* 31(1976), pp. 533–538.

BINNIE, C. A. "Bi-sensory Articulation Functions for Normal Hearing and Sensorineural Hearing Loss Patients," *Journal of the Academy of Rehabilitative Audiology*, 6(1973), pp. 43–53.

BINNIE, C. A. "Auditory-Visual Intelligibility of Various Speech Materials Presented in Three Noise Backgrounds," *Visual and Audio-visual Perception of Speech*, in H. B. Nielson and E. Kampp eds., Scandinavian Audiology, Supplement 4, 1974, pp. 255–280.

BINNIE, C. A. "Relevant Aural Rehabilitation," in *Hearing Disorders*, J. L. Northern ed, Boston: Little, Brown, 1976.

BINNIE, C. A., P. L. JACKSON, and A. A. MONTGOMERY, "Visual Intelligibility of Consonants: A Lipreading Screening Test with Implications for Aural Rehabilitation," *Journal of Speech and Hearing Disorders*, 41(1976), pp. 530–539.

BINNIE, C. A. "Effects of Age on the Visual Perception of Speech," in *Aural Rehabilitation for the Elderly*, M. Henoch ed., New York: Grune and Stratton, 1979, pp. 123–148.

BIRREN, J. E. *The Psychology of Aging.* Englewood Cliffs, New Jersey: Prentice-Hall, Inc., 1964.

BLUMENFELD, V. G., M. BERGMAN, and E. MILLER, "Speech Discrimination in an Aging Population", *Journal of Speech and Hearing Research*, 12 (1969), pp. 210–217.

BOOTHROYD, A. "Speech Perception and Sensorineural Hearing Loss," in *Auditory Management of Hearing Impaired Children*, Mark Ross and Thomas G. Giolas eds., Baltimore: University Park Press, 1978, pp. 117–144.

BOTWINICK, J., *Aging and Behavior*, New York: Springer, 1973.

BRUNT, M., "Prediction of Hearing Handicap With Staggered Spondaic Word Test." Paper presented at ASHA Convention, Atlanta, Georgia, 1979.

CARHART, R. "Hearing Aid Selection by University Clinics," *Journal of Speech and Hearing Research*, 15(1950), pp. 103–113.

CARHART, R. "Problems of the Hearing Impaired in Noisy Social Gatherings," in *Oto-Rhino-Laryngology: Proceedings of the Ninth International Congress* (Mexico), Amsterdam: Excerpta Medica, 1969, pp. 564–568.

CHALFANT J. C. and M. A. SCHEFFELIN, *Central Processing Dysfunctions in Children*, Bethesda, Maryland: U.S. Department of Health, Education and Welfare, 1969.

CHASSER, G. H. and T. G. GIOLAS "Normal Auditory Efficiency as Measured by the Hearing Performance Inventory," in *American Speech and Hearing Association Convention Program*, 1977, p. 176.

CHASSER, C. H. "Normal Auditory Efficiency as Measured by the Hearing Performance Inventory," Unpublished Manuscript, Storrs, Connecticut, Department of Communication Sciences, University of Connecticut, 1978.

COLE R. A. and B. SCOTT, "Towards Theory of Speech Perception," *Psychological Review*, 81(1974), pp. 348–374.

CRUM M. A. and T. W. TILLMAN, "Effects of Speaker-to-Noise Distance Upon Speech Intelligibility in Reverberation and Noise." Paper presented at American Speech and Hearing Association Convention, Detroit, Michigan, 1973.

DAVIS, H. "The Articulation Area and the Social Adequacy Index for Hearing," *The Laryngoscope,* 58(1948), pp. 761–778.

DAVIS, H. "Guidelines for Classification and Evaluation of Hearing Handicap in Relation to International Audiometric Zero," *Trans. American Academy of Ophthalmology and Otolaryngology,* 69(1965), pp. 740–751.

DAVIS H. and S. R. SILVERMAN, *Hearing and Deafness* (4th ed.), New York. Holt, Rhinehart and Winston, 1978.

DONAHUE, W. "Psychological aspects," in *The Care of the Geriatric Patient,* E. V. Cowdry and F. U. Steinberg eds., St. Louis, Missouri: Mosby Company, 1971.

EPSTEIN, A., T. G. GIOLAS, and E. OWENS, "Familiarity and Intelligibility of Mono-syllabic Word Lists," *Journal of Speech and Hearing Research,* 11(1968), pp. 435–438.

ERBER, N. P. "Auditory Detection of Spondaic Words in Wideband Noise by Adults with Normal Hearing and by Children with Profound Hearing Losses," *Journal of Speech and Hearing Research,* 14(1971a), pp. 372–381.

ERBER, N. P. "Auditory and Audiovisual Reception of Words in Low Frequency Noise by Children with Normal Hearing and by Children with Impaired Hearing," *Journal of Speech and Hearing Research,* 14(1971b), pp. 496–512.

ERBER, N. P. "Auditory, Visual and Auditory-Visual Recognition of Consonants by Children with Normal and Impaired Hearing," *Journal of Speech and Hearing Research,* 15(1972), pp. 413–422.

ERICKSON, J. G. *Speech Reading: An Aid to Communication,* Danville, Ill.: The Interstate Printers & Publishers, Inc., 1978.

EWERTSEN, H. W. and H. BIRK NIELSON, "A comparative Analysis of the Au-diovisual, Auditive and Visual Perception of Speech," *Acta Otolaryngologica,* 72(1971), pp. 201-205.

FARRIMOND, T. "Age Differences in the Ability to Use Visual Cues in Auditory Communication," *Language and Speech,* 2(1959), pp. 179–192.

FESTINGER, L. A., A theory of social comparison processes. Human Relations, Vol. 7, 1954.

FLANAGAN, J. C. "The Critical Incident Technique," *Psychological Bulletin,* 51(1954), pp. 327–358.

FLEMING, M. "A Total Approach to Communication Therapy," *Journal of the Academy of Rehabilitative Audiology,* V(1972), pp. 28–31.

FLETCHER, H. *Speech and Hearing in Communication.* New York. Van Nostrand, 1953.

FRENCH N. R. and J. C. STEINBERG, "Factors Governing the Intelligibility of Speech Sounds," *Journal of the Acoustical Society of America,* 19(1947), pp. 90–119.

GAETH, J. "A Study of Phonemic Regression Associated with Hearing Loss," disser-tation, Northwestern University, 1948.

GAY, T. "Effect of Filtering and Vowel Environment on Consonant Perception," *Journal of the Acoustical Society of America,* 48(1970), pp. 993–998.

GIOLAS, T. G. "Comparative Intelligibility Scores of Sentence Lists and Continuous Discourse," *Journal of Auditory Research,* 6(1966a), pp. 31–38.

GIOLAS, T. G. "Effectiveness of Social Adequacy Index," *Annals of Otology, Rhinology and Laryngology,* 75(1966b), pp. 1–6.

GIOLAS, T. G. "The Measurement of Hearing Handicap: A Point of View," *Maico Audiological Library Series,* 8(1970), pp. 20–23.

GIOLAS, T. G., H. S. COOKER, and J. R. DUFFY, "The Predictability of Words in Sentences," *Journal of Auditory Research,* 10(1970), pp. 328–334.

GIOLAS, T. G. and J. R. DUFFY, "Equivalency of CID and Revised CID Sentence Lists," *Journal of Speech and Hearing Research,* 16(1973), pp. 549–555.

GIOLAS, T. G. and A. EPSTEIN, "Comparative Intelligibility of Word Lists and Continuous Discourse," *Journal of Speech and Hearing Research,* 6(1963), pp. 349–358.

GIOLAS, T. G., E. OWENS, S. H. LAMB, and E. D. SCHUBERT, "Hearing Performance Inventory," *Journal of Speech and Hearing Disorders,* 44(1979), pp. 169–195.

GIOLAS, T. G. and D. J. WARK, "Communication Problems Associated with Unilateral Hearing Loss," *Journal of Speech and Hearing Disorders,* 32(1967), pp. 336–342.

GLORIG, A. and H. DAVIS, "Age, Noise and Hearing Loss," *Annals of Otology, Rhinology and Laryngology,* 70(1961), pp. 556–571.

GLORIG, A., D. WHEELER, R. QUIGGLE, W. GRINGS, and A. SUMMERFIELD, "1954 Wisconsin State Fair Hearing Survey," Monograph, *American Academy of Ophthalmology and Otolaryngology,* 1957.

GOETZINGER, C. P. "Word discrimination testing," in *Handbook of Clinical Audiology* (2nd ed.), Jack Katz ed., Baltimore: Williams and Wilkins 1978, pp. 149–158.

GOETZINGER, C., G. PROUD, D. DIRKS, and J. EMBREY, "A Study of Hearing in Advanced Age," *Archives of Otolaryngology,* 73(1961), pp. 662–674.

GOLDMAN, R., M. FRISTOE, and R. WOODCOCK, *The Goldman-Fristoe-Woodcock Test of Auditory Discrimination.* Circle Pines, Minnesota: American Guidance Service, 1970.

HARDICK, E. J. "Aural Rehabilitation Programs for the Aged Can be Successful," *Journal of Rehabilitative Audiology, (1977), pp. 51–67.*

HARDICK, E. J., H. J. OYER, and P. E. IRION, "Lipreading Performance as Related to Measurements of Vision," *Journal of Speech and Hearing Research,* 13(1970), pp. 92–100.

HARDICK, E. J., W. MELNICK, N. A. HAWES, J. P. PILLION, R. G. STEPHENS, and D. J. PERLMUTTER, "Compensation for Hearing Loss for Employees under Jurisdiction of the U.S. Department of Labor: Benefit Formula and Assessment Procedures," Final Report—Contract No. J-9-E-9-0205, Ohio State University, 1980.

HARFORD, E. and J. BARRY, "A Rehabilitative Approach to the Problem of Unilateral Hearing Impairment: Contralateral Routing of Signals (CROS)," *Journal of Speech and Hearing Disorders,* 30(1965), pp. 121–138.

HARFORD, E. and B. DODDS, "The Clinical Application of CROS," *Archives of Otolaryngology,* 83(1966), pp. 455–464.

HARRIS, J. D. "Pure Tone Acuity and the Intelligibility of Everyday Speech." *Journal of the Acoustical Society of America,* 37(1965), pp. 824–830.

HARRIS, J. D., J. D. HAINES, and C. K. MYERS, "The Importance of Hearing at 3Kc for Understanding Speeded Speech," *The Laryngoscope,* 70(1960), pp. 131–146.

HEATON, J. M. *The Eye: Phenomenology and Psychology of Function and Disorder.* London, England: Tavistock, 1968.

HIGH, W. S., G. FAIRBANKS, and A. GLORIG, "Scale of Self-Assessment of Hearing Handicap," *Journal of Speech and Hearing Disorders,* 29(1964), pp. 215–230.

HULL, R. H. *Hearing Impairment Among Aging Persons.* Lincoln, Nebraska: Cliffs Notes, Inc., 1977.

HUTTON, C, E. T. CURRAY, and M. B. ARMSTRONG, "Semi-Diagnostic Test Materials for Aural Rehabilitation," *Journal of Speech and Hearing Disorders,* 24(1959), pp. 318–329.

JERGER, J. "Diagnostic Audiometry, Chapter 3," in *Modern Developments in Audiology* (2nd Ed.), J. Jerger ed, New York: Academic Press, 1973a.

JERGER, J. "Audiological Findings in Aging," *Adv Oto-Rhino-Laryng,* 20(1973b), pp. 115–124.

JERGER, J., C. SPEAKS, and J. L. TRAMMEL, "A New Approach to Speech Audiometry," *Journal of Speech and Hearing Disorders,* 33(1968), pp. 318–328.

KALIKOW, D. N., K. N. STEVENS, and L. L. ELLIOT, "Development of a Test of Speech Intelligibility in Noise Using Sentence Material with Controlled Word Predictability," *Journal of the Acoustical Society of America,* 61(1977), pp. 1337–1351.

KALISH, R. A. *The Later Years: Social Applications of Gerontology.* Monterey, California: Brooks/Cole Publishing Company, 1977.

KELL, R. L., J. C. G. PEARSON, W. I. ACTON, and W. TAYLOR, "Social Effects of Hearing Loss Due to Weaving Noise," in *Occupational Hearing Loss,* D. W. Robinson ed., London, England: Academic Press, 1971, pp. 179–191.

KRYTER, K. D. "Hearing Impairment for Speech: Evaluation from Pure Tone Audiometry," *Archives of Otolaryngology,* 77(1963) pp. 598–602.

KRYTER, K. D. "Impairment to Hearing from Exposure to Noise." *Journal of the Acoustical Society of America,* 53(1973), pp. 1211–1234.

KULLER, J. N. "The relationships among self-assessment of hearing handicap, locas-of-control, and audiological measures of hearing impairment in presbycusic individuals." Unpublished Doctoral Dissertation, New York University, 1976.

LIBERMAN, A. M., F. S. COOPER, D. P. SHANKWEILER, and M. STUDDERT-KENNEDY, "Perception of the Speech Code," *Psychological Review,* 74(1967), pp. 431–461.

LIPSCOMB, D. M. "Noise in the Environment: The Problem," *Maico Audiological Library Series,* 8(1970), pp. 1–6.

LLOYD, L. L. "The Audiologic Assessment of Deaf Students," in The Proceedings of the 45th Meeting of the Convention of the American Instructors of the Deaf, Washington, D.C.: U.S. Government Printing Office, 1972, pp. 585–594.

**Lochner, J. P. A. and J. F. Burger,** "The Influence of Reflections on Auditorium Acoustics," *Journal of Sound Vibration,* 1(1964), pp. 426–454.

**Lovering, L. J. and E. J. Hardick,** "Lipreading Performance as a Function of Visual Acuity," paper presented at the Annual Meeting of the American Speech and Hearing Association, Chicago, Illinois, 1969.

**Macrae, J.** "A Procedure for Classifying Degree of Hearing Loss," *Journal of the Otolaryngological Society of Australia,* 1(1976), pp. 26–35.

**Martin, F. N.** *Introduction to Audiology,* Second edition, Englewood Cliffs, New Jersey: Prentice Hall, 1981.

**McCartney, J. H., Maurer, J. F., and Sorenson, F. D.** "A Comparison of the Handicap Scale and the Hearing Measurement Scale with Standard Audiometric Measures on a Geriatric Population." *Journal of Auditory Research,* 16 (1976), pp. 51–58.

**McNeil, M. and J. G. Alpiner,** "A Study of the Reliability of the Denver Scale of Communication Function," unpublished study, University of Denver, 1975.

**McReynolds, L. V.** "The Impractibility of Diagnostic Categories to the Treatment of Language Impaired Children," *ASHA Bulletin,* 11(1967), pp. 4–14.

**Mead, B.** "Emotional Struggles in Adjusting to Old Age," *Post Grad Med,* 31(1962), pp. 156–160.

**Miller, G. A.** "The Masking of Speech," *Psychological Bulletin,* 44(1947), pp. 105–129.

**Miller, G. A.** *Language and Communication.* New York: McGraw-Hill, 1951.

**Miller, G. A., G. A. Heise, and W. Lichten,** "The Intelligibility of Speech as a Function of the Context of Test Materials," *Journal of Experimental Psychology,* 41(1951), pp. 329–335.

**Miller, G. A. and P. E. Nicely,** "An Analysis of Perceptual Confusions Among Some English Consonants," *Journal of the Acoustical Society of America,* 27(1955), pp. 338–352.

**Nabelek, A. K. and J. M. Pickett,** "Reception of Consonants in a Classroom as Affected by Monaural and Binaural Listening, Noise Reverberation and Hearing Aids," *Journal of the Acoustical Society of America,* 56(1974a), pp. 628–639.

**Nabelek A. K. and J. M. PICKETT,** "Monaural and Binaural Speech Perception Through Hearing Aids Under Noise and Reverberation with Normal and Hearing-Impaired Listeners," *Journal of Speech and Hearing Research,* 17(1974b), pp. 724–739.

**Nett, E. M., L. G. Doefler, and J. Matthews,** "The Relationship Between Audiological Measures and Handicap," unpublished manuscript, Vocational Rehabilitation Administration, Project No. 167, 1960.

**Noble, W. G.** "A New Concept of Damage Risk Criterion," *Annals of Occupational Hygiene,* 13(1970), pp. 69–70.

**Noble, W. G.** *Assessment of the Hearing Impaired. A Critique and a New Method.* New York: Academic Press, 1978.

**Noble, W. G. and G. R. C. Atherley,** "The Hearing Measurement Scale: A Questionaire for the Assessment of Auditory Disability," *Journal of Auditory Research,* 10(1970), pp. 229–250.

OLSEN, W. O. and R. CARHART, "Development of Test Procedures for Evaluation of Monaural Hearing Aids," *Bulletin of Prosthetic Research,* 10(1967), pp. 22–49.

OLSEN, W. O. and T. W. TILLMAN, "Hearing Aids and Sensorineural Hearing Loss," *Annals of Otology, Rhinology and Laryngology,* 77(1968), pp. 717–726.

OWENS, E., M. BENEDICT, and E. D. SCHUBERT, "Consonant Phonemic Errors Associated with Pure-Tone Configurations and Certain Kinds of Hearing Impairment," *Journal of Speech and Hearing Research,* 15(1972), pp. 308–322.

OWENS, E. and S. FUJIKAWA, "The H.P.I. and Hearing Aid Use in Profound Hearing Loss," *Journal of Speech and Hearing Disorders,* 23(1980), pp. 470–479.

OWENS, E. and E. D. SCHUBERT, "The Development of Consonant Items for Speech Discrimination Testing," *Journal of Speech and Hearing Research,* 11(1968a), pp. 656–667.

OWENS, E., C. B. TALBOTT, and E. D. SCHUBERT, "Vowel Discrimination of Hearing Impaired Listeners," *Journal of Speech and Hearing Research,* 11(1968b), pp. 649–655

OYER, W. and M. DOUDNA, "Structural Analysis of Word Responses Made by Hard-of-hearing Subjects on a Discrimination Test," *Archives of Otolaryngology,* 70(1959), pp. 357–364.

PELSON, R. O. and W. F. PRATHER, "Effects of Visual Message-Related Cues, Age and Hearing Impairment on Speechreading Performance," *Journal of Speech and Hearing Research,* 17(1974), pp. 518–525.

PETERS, G. M. "The Relationship Between Some Measures of Hearing Loss and Self-assessment of Hearing Handicap," Unpublished Doctoral Dissertation, Wayne State University, Detroit, Michigan, 1974.

RAMSDELL, O. A. "The Psychology of the Hard-of-Hearing and the Deafened Adult," in *Hearing and Deafness* (4th ed.), H. Davis and S. R. Silverman eds., New York: Holt, Rhinehart and Winston, 1978.

RESNICK D. M. and M. H. BECKER, "Hearing Aid Evaluation—A New Approach," *Asha,* 5(1963), pp. 695–699.

ROSEN, J. K. "Psychological and Social Aspects of the Evaluation of Acquired Hearing Impairment," *Audiology,* 18(1979), pp. 238–252.

ROSENZWEIG M. R. and L. POSTMAN, "Frequency of Usage and the Perception of Words," *Science,* 127(1958), pp. 263–266.

ROSS, M. "Classroom Acoustics and Speech Intelligibility," in *Handbook of Clinical Audiology,* J. Katz ed., Baltimore: Williams and Wilkins, 1978, pp. 469–498.

ROSS, M., R. J. DUFFY, H. S. COOKER, and R. L. SARGEANT, "Contribution of the Lower Audible Frequencies to the Recognition of Emotions," *American Anals of the Deaf,* 118(1973), pp. 37–42.

ROSS, M., M. KESSLER, M. PHILLIPS, and J. LERMAN, "Visual, Auditory and Combined Mode Presentations of the WIPI Test to Hearing-Impaired Children," *Volt Review,* 74(1972), pp. 90–96.

ROUSEY, C. "Psychological Reactions to Hearing Loss," *Journal of Speech and Hearing Disorders,* 36(1971), pp. 382–389.

SANDERS, D. A. "Hearing Aid Orientation and Counseling," in *Amplification for the Hearing-Impaired,* M. Pollack ed., New York: Grune and Stratton, 1980.

SATALOFF, J., L. VASSALO, and H. MENDUKE, "Presbycusis: Air- and Bone-Conduction Thresholds," *Laryngoscope*, 75(1965), pp. 889–901.

SCHER A. E. and E. OWENS, "Consonant Confusions Associated with Hearing Loss Above 2000 Hz," *Journal of Speech and Hearing Research*, 17(1964), pp. 669–681.

SCHO, R. L. and TANNAHILL, J. C. "Hearing Handicap Scores and Categories for Subjects with Normal and Impaired Hearing Sensitivity," *Journal of the American Auditory Society*, 3 (1977), pp. 134–139.

SCHUKNECHT, H. "Further Observations on the Pathology of Presbycusis," *Archives of Otolaryngology*, 80(1964), pp. 369–382.

SCHUKNECHT, H. *Pathology of the Ear.* Cambridge, Massachusetts: Harvard University Press, 1974.

SCHULTZ, M. C. "Suggested Improvements in Speech Discrimination Testing." *Journal of Auditory Research*, 4(1964), pp. 1–14.

SHOOP, C., and C. A. BINNIE, "The Effect of Age on the Visual Perception of Speech," *Scandinavian Audiology*, 7(1978).

SHORE, I., R. C. BILGER, and I. J. HIRSCH, "Hearing Aid Evaluation: Reliability of Repeated Measurements, *Journal of Speech and Hearing Disorders*, 25(1960), pp. 152–170.

SHOSTROM E. L., *Man the Manipulator.* Nashville, Tennessee: Abingdon Press, 1967.

SILVERMAN S. R. and D. CALVERT, "Conservation and Development of Speech," in *Hearing and Deafness* (4th ed.), H. Davis and S. R. Silverman eds., New York: Holt, Rhinehart and Winston, 1978.

SILVERMAN S. R. and I. J. HIRSCH, "Problems Related to the Use of Speech in Clinical Audiometry." *Annals of Otology, Rhinology and Laryngology*, 64(1955), pp. 1234–1244.

SILVERMAN S. R., W. R. THURLOW, T. E. WALSH, and H. DAVIS, "Improvement in the Social Adequacy of Hearing Following the Fenestration Operation," *The Laryngoscope*, 58(1948), pp. 607–631.

SIMPSON, R. H. "Stability in the Meanings for Quantitative Terms: A Comparison Over 20 Years," *Quarterly Journal of Speech*, 49(1963), pp. 146–151.

SPEAKS C. and J. JERGER, "Method for Measurement of Speech Identification," *Journal of Speech and Hearing Research*, 8(1965), pp. 185–194.

SPEAKS, C., J. JERGER, and J. TRAMMELL, "Measurement of Hearing Handicap," *Journal of Speech and Hearing Research*, 134(1970), pp. 768–776.

SUTTER, A. "The Ability of Mildly Hearing-Impaired Individuals to Discriminate Speech in Noise," Dissertation, University of Maryland, 1977.

TANNAHILL, J. C. "The Hearing Handicap Scale as a Measure of Hearing and Benefit," *Journal of Speech and Hearing Disorders*, 44(1976), pp. 91–99.

TILLMAN, T. W. and R. CARHART, "An Expanded Test for Speech Discrimination Utilizing CNC Monosyllabic Words (N.U. Auditory Test No. 6)," Technical Report No. SAM TR 66–55, U.S.A.F. School of Aerospace Medicine, Brooks Air Force Base, Texas, 1966.

TILLMAN, T. W. and J. JERGER, "Some Factors Affecting the Spondee Threshold in Normal Hearing Subjects," *Journal of Speech and Hearing Research*, 2(1959), pp. 141–146.

TILLMAN, T. W., R. CARHART, and W. O. OLSEN, "Hearing Aid Efficiency in a Competing Speech Situation," *Journal of Speech and Hearing Research,* 13(1974), pp. 789–811.

VERNON, M. "Sociological and Psychological Factors Associated with Hearing Loss," *Journal of Speech and Hearing Research,* 12(1969), pp. 541–563.

WEBSTER, E. J. *Counselling with Parents of Handicapped Children: Guidelines for Improving Communication,* New York: Grune and Stratton, 1977.

WEALE, R. A. "On the Eye," in *Behavior, Aging, and the Nervous System,* A. T. Welford and J. E. Birren eds., Springfield, Illinois: Charles C Thomas, 1965.

WILLEFORD, J. A. "The Geriatric Patient," in *Audiological Assessment,* D. Rose ed., Englewood Cliffs, New Jersey: Prentice-Hall, Inc., 1971.

ZARNOCH, J. M. and J. G. ALPINER, "The Denver Scale of Communication Function for Senior Citizens Living in Retirement Centers," unpublished study, 1977.